MW01633917

DISEASES CAUSED BY MASTURBATION

OR, ONANISM

DR. SAMUEL-AUGUSTE TISSOT

—

With an Introduction by C.V. Ruisdael

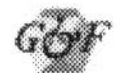

GOTTFRIED & FRITZ
Philadelphia & New York

 Published in the United States by Gottfried & Fritz, Inc., New York & Philadelphia.

ISBN : 978-0-9861772-1-7

www.gottfriedandfritz.com

Manufactured in the United States of America.

Editor's Introduction

On the Diseases Caused by Masturbation, which Samuel-Auguste Tissot originally published in 1760 under the French title, *L'Onanism. Dissertation sur les maladies produites par la masturbation*, is a medical treatise on the ill effects of masturbation on both the mind and the body. The book recounts stories from his own patients and from the patients of other renowned European doctors to support his claim that masturbation is deleterious to a person's body and mind. Tissot also uses quotes from the ancient physicians, such as Galen and Celsus, as well as the most noted doctors of his day, such as Herman Boerhaave, to further strengthen his claim.

One of the physicians whom Tissot quotes claims, for example, that masturbation causes "young persons [to] assume the air and the diseases of the aged; they become pale, stupid, effeminate, idle, weak, and even void of understanding; their bodies bend forward, their legs are weak, they have a disgust for every thing, become fit for nothing, and many are affected with paralysis"; and another, that "the too great loss of semen produces weakness, debility, immobility, convulsions, emaciation, dryness, pains in the membranes of the brain, impairs the senses, particularly that of sight, gives rise to dorsal consumption, indolence, and to the several diseases connected with them." And Tissot himself writes of one of his own patients, "A young man, not sixteen years old, became addicted to masturbation to so great a degree, that finally, instead of semen there was an emission of blood, which was followed by excessive pain and inflammation of all the genital organs." However, the reader should not mistake this piece as an out-moded medicinal work; Tissot also summarizes the beliefs of some ancient philosophers on masturbation and its effects on the mind. "Epicurus," he writes, "regarded the semen as a *part* of the *soul* and *body* and prescribed rules for carefully preserving it."

Tissot himself was born in Grancy, Switzerland in 1728, but practiced for most of his life in the Swiss city of Lausanne. He was one of the most notable physicians of his day. He was appointed Vatican medical advisor and once even received a letter of praise from Napoleon Bonaparte, who commended him in a letter dated 1 April 1787, for his, "days in treating humanity," and even conceded that Tissot's fame and reputation "has reached even into the mountains of Corsica." Bonaparte then concluded, that he has a great deal of "respect for [Tissot's] works." And Bonaparte was not mistaken in his admiration of Tissot; even modern doctors still regard him as a basis for "future generations of doctors." (*Journal of Neurology, Volume 233, Number 2.*)

Tissot is most noted in the medical community for a chapter that he wrote on the migraine in his more comprehensive *Traité des nerfs et de leurs maladies* (*Treatise on the Nerves and Nervous Disorders*) and modern doctors now regard him as "the classical authority on the migraine." But Tissot's best-seller, and one of the best-selling medical books in the entire 18th century, was a small book that he published in 1761 entitled, *Avis au peuple sur sa santé* (*Advice to People on their Health*). As the title suggests, Tissot's best-seller was a handbook for people who wanted to maintain good health and establish habits that were essential to living long and healthy lives.

One year before Tissot had published his famous *Avis au peuple sa santé*, he published the following work: *L'Onanism: Dissertation sur les maladies produites par la masturbation* (*Onanism: A Dissertation on the Diseases Caused by Masturbation*).

He continued to practice in Lausanne until his death in 1797 at the age of 69.

CONTENTS

DISEASES CAUSED BY MASTURBATION

Introduction

—

Our bodies are constantly wasting; and if this waste were not repaired we should soon become extremely weak. This reparation is effected by food; the food undergoes successive changes in the body, which are termed nutrition. Whether this does, or does not take place, the food becomes useless, and will not prevent us from being affected with all the evils produced by exhaustion. Of all the causes which prevent nutrition, there is none more common than too abundant evacuations.

Our bodies, and those of animals generally, are so constructed that in order for the aliment to acquire the degree of preparation necessary to nourish them, a certain quantity of the fluids, which are perfect or naturalized, if we may use the expression, are necessary. If these do not exist, digestion is imperfect, in proportion to the importance of the fluid deficient.

A robust nurse, who would be destroyed by the loss of a few pounds of blood in a single day, may supply the same quantity of milk to her child, several days in succession, without being sensibly incommoded by it; because of all the fluids, the milk is the least assimilated; it is a fluid almost foreign to the body, while the blood is essential. There is another, the seminal fluid, which has so much influence on the strength of the body and on the perfection of digestion which restores it, that physicians of every age have unanimously admitted, that the loss of one ounce of it, enfeebles more than forty ounces of blood. We may form some idea of its importance by observing the effects it produces; when it begins to form, the voice, the countenance, and even the features change; the beard grows, and the whole body often assumes another appearance, since the muscles become so large and firm that they form a sensible difference between the body of an adult, and that of one who has not arrived at puberty. All these developments are prevented by debilitating the organ which serves to separate the fluid producing them. Correct observations prove that the extirpation of the testicles, at the period of virility, causes the loss of the beard, and the return of an infantile voice. Can we doubt, after this of its action on the whole body, and not perceive the many bad consequences with which the emission of so precious a fluid must be attended. Its destination determines the only legitimate mode of its evacuation. It is sometimes emitted in diseases. It may also be discharged involuntarily, during libidinous dreams. The author of Genesis[1] has left us the history of the crime of Onan[2], doubtless to mention his punishment; and we learn from Galen[3], that Diogenes[4] was guilty of the same crime.

If the dangerous consequences arising from the too abundant discharge of semen, depended only on the quantity, or were the same under different modes of evacuation, the quantities in each being equal, then it would be of little importance, physically speaking, in which it took place. But there is a difference; a too great quantity of semen lost in the natural way, causes very serious symptoms, but these are much more serious when the same amount has been discharged by unnatural means. The diseases of those exhausted by natural connections, are terrible; but those produced by onanism, are much more so. The last are, properly speaking, the object of this work, but they are connected so intimately with the first, that they cannot well be separated. The description of them in common will form the first article; in the second, we shall explain the causes, together with those which render masturbation more dangerous; the mode of cure, and remarks on some analogous diseases, will terminate the work. Some observations of the best authors will occasionally be added.

ARTICLE I.

SYMPTOMS.

SECTION I.

DESCRIPTION OF THE DISEASE TAKEN FROM MEDICAL WORKS.

Hippocrates, the oldest and most correct observer, has already described the diseases produced by abusing the pleasures of venery, under the term, *dorsal consumption.* "This disease," says he, "arises from the dorsal portion of the spinal marrow. It principally attacks young married people, or the licentious. They have no fever, and although they eat well, they grow thin and waste away. They have a sensation of ants crawling from the head down along the spine. Whenever they go to stool, or evacuate their urine, a considerable quantity of very thin seminal fluid escapes from the urethra. They lose the powers of procreation, yet often dream of venereal pleasures. They become very weak, and walking produces shortness of breath; they have pains in the head and ringing in the ears; finally an acute *fever* (*Libiria*) supervenes and they die." We shall mention this fever in another place.

Some physicians have ascribed to the same cause, a disease which he has described, in another place, and have termed it the *second dorsal consumption of Hippocrates*, and which has some relation to the first. But the preservation of the strength which he mentions particularly, seems to us a conclusive proof, that this disease does not depend on the same cause, but seems rather to be a rheumatic affection.

"These pleasures," says Celsus[5], in his excellent work on the preservation of health, "are always injurious to weak persons, and their abuse prostrates the strength." We can find nothing more frightful, than the description, by Aretæus[6], of the diseases produced by a too abundant evacuation of semen. "Young persons assume the air and the diseases of the aged; they become pale, stupid, effeminate, idle, weak, and even void of understanding; their bodies bend forward, their legs are weak, they have a disgust for every thing, become fit for nothing, and many are affected with paralysis." In another place, he mentions the abuse of these pleasures among the six causes which produce paralysis.

Galen has seen diseases of the brain and nerves from the same cause, and the powers of the body impaired; and he also relates that a man who was convalescent from a violent attack of disease, died the same night after coition with his wife.

Pliny, the naturalist, informs us that Cornelius Gallus, the old pretor, and Titus Etherius, a Roman knight, died in the act of copulation.

Aetius says "the stomach is deranged, all the body wastes, becomes pale, dry, and the eyes sunken." These remarks of the most respectable ancient writers are confirmed by the moderns. Sanctorius who has examined, with the utmost care, all the causes which act on our bodies, has observed, that this weakens the stomach, destroys digestion, prevents insensible perspiration, the derangements of which produce such evil consequences, disposes to calculous diseases, diminishes the natural warmth, and is usually attended with a loss, or derangement of sight.

Lomnius, in his fine commentaries on the passages of Celsus whom we have just cited, supports the remarks of the author by his own observations. "Frequent emissions of semen relax, weaken, dry, enervate the body, and produce numerous other evils, as apoplexies, lethargies, epilepsies, loss of sight, trembling, paralysis, and all kinds of painful affections."

One cannot read without horror the description left us by Tulpius, the celebrated burgomaster[7] and physician of Amsterdam. "Not only," says he, "the spinal marrow wastes, but the whole body and mind becomes languid, and the patient perishes in misery. Samuel Vespertius was attacked first with a humor upon the back of his neck and head; it then passed to the spine, to the loins, to the lower and lateral region of the abdomen, and to the hips; this unhappy man was affected with so much pain, that he was entirely disfigured, and was emaciated so gradually by a slow fever, that he more than once asked to be relieved from his misery by death."

Nothing says a celebrated physician of Luvain, weakens the system so much.

Blancard has known simple gonorrheas, dropsies, and consumptions, to depend on this cause; and Muys has seen a man of good age attacked with spontaneous gangrene, of the foot, which he attributed to the same kind of excesses.

In the *Mémoires des curieux de la nature*[8] is mentioned a case of blindness: it deserves to be given at length. "We are ignorant," says the author, "what sympathy the testicles have with the body, but particularly with the eyes." Salmuth has known a sensible hypochondriac to become a fool, and in another man the brain to be so collapsed that it was heard to rattle in the cranium, both from excesses in venery. I have known myself a man, fifty-nine years of age, who, three weeks after marrying a young wife, became blind, and in four months died.

"The too great loss of the animal spirits weakens the stomach and destroys the appetite; and nutrition not taking place, the action of the heart becomes more feeble; all parts languish, and the patient becomes epileptic." It is true we are ignorant whether the animal spirits and the seminal fluid are the same; but observations show, as we shall see hereafter, that these two fluids are very analogous, and that loss of one or the other, produces the same complaints. Hoffman has seen the most frightful symptoms ensue from the loss of semen. "After long nocturnal pollutions," says he, "the patient not only loses strength, becomes emaciated and pale, but the memory is impaired, a continual sensation of coldness affects all the extremities, the sight becomes dim, the voice harsh, and the whole body, gradually wasted ; the sleep is disturbed by unpleasant dreams, does not refresh, and pains are felt like those produced by bruises."

In a consultation for a young man who, among other diseases produced by masturbation, was affected with weakness in the eyes, he says, I have seen several instances of young men who, at mature age, when the body possesses all its strength, were attacked, not only with severe pain and redness of the eyes, but the sight became so feeble that they could neither read nor write." He adds, "I have even seen two cases of *gutta serena* from the same cause." The history of the disorder which gave rise to this consultation will be read with interest. "A young man commenced masturbation, when fifteen years old, and having indulged in it till he was twenty three, experienced so great feebleness in his head and eyes, that during the emission of semen there was severe pain in the latter. When he attempted to read any thing he had a feeling similar to that of drunkenness; the pupil was extraordinarily dilated; the eyes were exceedingly painful; the eyelids very heavy, and glued together every night; they were often filled with tears, and a whitish matter collected very abundantly in the two corners which were very painful. Although he ate with a good appetite, still he was extremely emaciated; and after he had taken food, appeared as if drunk." The same author has mentioned another case of which he was an eyewitness and which we think proper to mention here. "A young man, eighteen years old, who had had frequent connections with a servant girl, suddenly fainted and trembled exceedingly in all his extremities; his countenance was red, and his pulse very small. He recovered from this state at the end of an hour, but continued very feeble. The same phenomena occurred very frequently with severe pain, and at the end of eight days there was a contraction and tumor in the right arm with a pain in the elbow, which was always increased during the paroxysm. The disease increased for some time, but was finally cured by Hoffman."

Boerhaave[9] portrays these diseases in that masterly manner and with that precision which characterize all his descriptions. "The too great loss of semen produces weakness, debility, immobility, convulsions, emaciation, dryness, pains in the membranes of the brain, impairs the senses, particularly that of sight, gives rise to dorsal consumption, indolence, and to the several diseases connected with them."

The cases, narrated by this great man to his auditors in explaining to them this aphorism, which related to the different kinds of evacuations, ought not to be omitted. "I have seen," says he, "a sick man where the disease commenced by a lassitudes and feebleness in the body, particularly in the loins: it was accompanied by twitching of the tendons, periodical spasms and loss of flesh, so as to destroy the whole body; also pains in the membranes of the cerebrum, pains which the patient terms (*ardeur sèche*) *a dry burning*, which constantly inflames this most noble organ."

"I have also seen one young man affected with dorsal consumption. His figure was good; and although often cautioned against indulging in these pleasures, he did not regard it, and became so deformed before death, that the layer of flesh which appears above the spinous processes of the lumbar vertebra, entirely disappeared. The cerebrum in this case seemed to be consumed; in fact, the patient seemed to be stupid, and became so stiff, that we have never seen the body so immovable from any other cause. The eyes are so dull that the sight is nearly lost."

De Senac mentions in the first edition of his *Essays*, the dangers attending masturbation, and states that all who indulge in this vice will be affected in the flower of their youth with the infirmities of age. We can see in the following editions why this and other remarks of the same character were suppressed.

Ludwig, in describing the diseases resulting from too frequent evacuations, does not forget that of the semen. "Young people of both sexes, who indulge in lasciviousness, ruin their health by wasting strength which was designed to make them vigorous, and finally fall into consumption."

De Gotter details the sad accidents arising from this cause; but they are too long to copy. We refer to the work all those who can read the language in which it is written.

Van Swieten, after quoting the description of Hippocrates mentioned above, adds, "I have seen all these symptoms, and several others, in those unfortunate people who indulged in self-pollutions. I have employed uselessly, for three years, all the resources of medicine, for a young man who was diseased in consequence of this practice with wandering, frightful, and general pains, with a sensation sometimes of heat, and sometimes of cold, in every part of the body, but particularly in the loins. Afterwards these pains having diminished, his thighs and legs were so cold, that although they seemed of the natural temperature when touched, he was constantly warming himself by the fire, even during the warmest days of summer. I noticed particularly, all this time, a continual rotatory motion of the testicles in the scrotum, and the patient felt a similar motion in the loins." This account does not mention whether this unfortunate creature died in three years or continued to languish sometime longer which would be more dreadful; he could not have recovered.

Kloekof, in a very fine work on the diseases of the mind which depend on the body, confirms by his observations what we have already mentioned. "A too great loss of semen weakens all the solid parts; hence arise weakness, idleness, phthisis, tabes dorsalis, stupidity, affections of the senses, faintings and convulsions."

Hoffman had already remarked that those young people who practice the infamous habit of masturbation, lose gradually all the faculties of the mind, particularly the memory, and become entirely unfit for study.

Levis describes all these symptoms. We shall translate from his work only what relates to the mind. "All the symptoms which arise from excesses of females, follow still more promptly, and in youth, the abominable practice of masturbation, and it is difficult to paint them in as frightful colors as they deserve: young persons addict themselves to this practice without knowing the enormity of the crime, and all the consequences which physically result from it. The mind is affected by all the diseases of the body, but particularly by those arising from this cause. The most dismal melancholy, indifference, and aversion to all pleasures, the impossibility to take part in conversation, the sense of their own misery, the consciousness of having brought it upon themselves, the necessity of renouncing the happiness of marriage, all affect them so much that they renounce the world—blessed if they escape suicide."

Cases hereafter to be mentioned will confirm this frightful picture. That of Storcq in his fine work, the history of the treatment of diseases, is no less terrible; but we refer to the work itself, which no physician should pass unnoticed.

Before proceeding to the cases which have been communicated to us, we shall terminate this section by a fine passage from Gaubius. He not only mentions the symptoms, but indicates the causes, with that force, truth, sagacity, and exactness, which belong only to the great masters. It is a valuable description, the power of which cannot be preserved in a translation. "Immoderata seminis profusio, non solum utilissimi humoris jactura, sed ipso etiam motu convulsivo, quo emittitur, frequentius repetito, imprimis lædit. Etenim summam voluptatem universalis excipit virium resolutio, quæ crebro ferri nequit, quin enervet. Collatoria autem corporis quo magis emulgentur, eo plus homorum aliunde ad se trahunt, succisque sic ad genitalia derivatis, reliquæ partes depauperantur. Inde ex nimia venere, lassitudo, debilitas, immobilitas, incessus, de lumbis ; encephali dolores, convulsiones sensuum omnium, maxime visus, habitudo, cæcitas, fatuitas, circulatio febrilis, exsiccatio, macies, tabes et pulmonica et dorsalis effeminatio. Augentur hæc mala atque insanabilia fiunt ob perpetuum in venerem pruritum, quem mens, non minus quam corpus, tandem contrahit, quoque efficitur, ut et dormientes obscena phantasmata exerceant, et in tentiginem pronæ partes quavis occasione impetum concipiant onerique et stimulo fit quam libet exigua reparati spermatis copia levissimo conatu, et vel fine hoc, de relaxatis loculis relapsura. Quocirca liquet, quare adolescentia florem adeo pessundet iste excessus."

SECTION II.

CASES COMMUNICATED.

We shall follow the order in which the cases were received. I have seen, says my illustrious friend Zimmerman, a man twenty-three years of age, who became epileptic, after having weakened his body by frequent masturbations. Whenever he had nocturnal pollutions, a perfect epileptic fit succeeded. The same thing happened after masturbation, from which he did not abstain, notwithstanding the symptoms, and all that was said to him. When the fit had passed, he felt acute pains in the kidneys and around the coccyx[10]. Having discontinued this practice for some time, I cured him of the nocturnal emissions, and I hoped even to arrest the epilepsy, the fits of which had already disappeared. His strength, appetite, sleep, and fine color returned, although he previously resembled a cadaver. But having again returned to his masturbations, which were always followed by an attack, he finally had fits, even in the streets, and was found dead one morning in his chamber, having fallen from his bed, and bathed in blood. A question presented itself to me, when I read this case; are those who commit suicide, more guilty than this person?

Without entering into details, my friend adds that he knows another in the same situation. I have since learned that it terminated in the same manner. I have known, says Zimmerman, a man of fine talents, and almost universal knowledge, the activity of whose mind was destroyed by frequent pollutions, and whose body was in the state of that patient who consulted Boerhaave, and which we shall mention in another place.

The next two facts were communicated by Rast, jun., the celebrated physician at Lyons, with whom I had the pleasure of passing some months at Montpelier. A young man of Montpelier, a student of medicine, died from excesses of this kind. The idea of his crime had so affected his mind, that he died in a kind of despair, and fancied he saw hell open at his side, ready to receive him. A child of this city, six or seven years old, taught, I believe, by a servant girl, polluted himself so often that the slow fever which supervened soon destroyed him. His desire for the commission of this act was so great, that he could not be prevented during the last few days of his life. When told that he hastened his death, he consoled himself by saying he should the sooner meet his father, who died some months previously.

Miege, the celebrated physician of Basle, known in the literary world by his excellent dissertations, and to whom his country is indebted for vaccination, which he continues with much success, has communicated a letter from Professor Stehelin, a name dear to literature, in which we have found some useful and interesting observations. I have reserved some for the latter part of this work, where they will be more in place.

The son of M. ———, aged fourteen or fifteen years, died of convulsions, in a kind of epilepsy, which arose solely from masturbation; he was treated without effect by the physicians of this city. I know a young lady twelve or thirteen years of age, who, from this detestable practice, has the appearance of being in a confirmed consumption, with a large and tense abdomen, fluor albus, and incontinence of urine. Although her case has been relieved by remedies, yet she continues in a languid state, and we are fearful of fatal consequences.

SECTION III.

DESCRIPTION OF THE DISEASE FROM AN ENGLISH WORK ENTITLED ONANIA.

Since the publication of this work, I have learned through the most respectable medium, that we ought not to believe all the cases mentioned in the English treatise, and that for this reason, and for some calumnies and obscenities, the German translation has been prohibited in the empire, by the exercise of the royal prerogative. For these reasons, we would have suppressed all our extracts from it; but for other considerations which we shall mention, they are retained with this caution. 1. Some of these objections relate only to the German edition. 2. Although some are only supposed facts, and others appear to have this character, yet most of them are too true. Finally, a third consideration which has influenced us is found in the letter of Stehelin. He says, I have received a letter from Hoffman of Maestricht, in which he remarks that he has treated unsuccessfully a person addicted to masturbation which had produced dorsal consumption, who was cured by the remedies mentioned in *Onania*[11], written by Dr. Bekkers, of London; this person afterwards became very corpulent and has now four children.

The English treatise, *Onania* is truly a chaos, the most unfinished work written for a long time. Only the cases can be read, for the reflections of the author are but theological and moral frivolities. I shall quote from this work, which is very long, only a sketch of the most common symptoms; the vivacity, the energetic expression of grief and of repentance in a few of the letters, and which are not found in the extracts, ought not to diminish the impression of horror which is felt on reading them, because this impression is founded on facts; and readers will be obliged to me for dispensing with a great number of letters without interest. I shall include under six heads all the symptoms, commencing with the most important, those of the mind.

1. All the intellectual faculties are enfeebled, the memory is destroyed, and sometimes the patients becomes slightly deranged; they have constantly mental inquietude, and their consciences reproach them so severely, that they often weep. They are subject to vertigo; all their senses, and particularly their sight and hearing, are impaired; their sleep, if they get any, is disturbed with frightful dreams.

2. The powers of the body fail entirely; the growth of those addicted to this habit before they arrive at maturity, is considerably deranged. Some do not sleep at all; others are constantly drowsy. Almost all have hypochondriasis[12] or hysteria and are afflicted with all the symptoms which supervene in these diseases; sadness, sighing, weeping, palpitations, dyspnoea[13], and debility. Some eat calcareous substances. Cough, slow fever, and consumption are the consequences of this practice in others.

3. The most acute pains also supervene; one complains of the head, another of the chest, stomach, intestines, rheumatic pains of the limbs, and tenderness on the slightest pressure in every part of the body.

4. Pimples not only appear on the face, (these are very common,) suppurating pustules are also seen on this part, around the nose, on the chest, and thighs, and large sloughs exist in different parts of the body. One of these patients complained of fleshy excrescence on his forehead.

5. The organs of generation are also affected in the diseases of which the sympathy of these parts is the first cause. Many are unable to produce an erection of the penis; in some emissions take place at the slightest erection or when at stool. A number are attacked with habitual gonorrhoea which debilitates, and the discharge often resembles a fetid sanies, or a saltish mucus; others are tormented with painful priapisms[14]. Dysuria strangury (*ardor urinæ*), cause great suffering in some patients, others again are affected with painful swellings in the testicles, the penis, the bladder, the spermatic cord. Finally, the impossibility of coition, or the vitiation of the semen, render sterile almost all those long addicted to this vice.

6. Most of the functions of the intestines are deranged; some patients complain of obstinate constipation, others of hemorrhoids or of a discharge of fetid matter from the anus. This last case resembles the young man mentioned by Hoffman, who after each masturbation was attacked with diarrhea, another cause of debility.

SECTION IV.

CASES BY THE AUTHOR.

The description of the first case which I shall give is shocking; I was frightened the first time I saw this unfortunate patient. I then felt more than ever, the necessity of mentioning to young people all the horrors of that abyss of misery into which they voluntarily plunge themselves. L. D——, a watchmaker, had been chaste and had enjoyed good health till he was seventeen years of age, when he became addicted to masturbation which was repeated once and often three times every day; the emission of semen was always preceded and attended by a slight loss of consciousness, and a convulsive action of the extensor muscles of the head, which drew it strongly backward, while the neck was very much swelled. One year had not elapsed, until he began to feel very weak after each act of masturbation; this was not sufficient to arrest his progress in this vice; his mind, already entirely absorbed in the commission of these acts, was incapable of other thoughts; repetitions became more frequent every day, till at length, he found himself in a very dangerous situation. Wise too late, the disease had already made such progress that he could not be cured; the genital organs had become so irritable and weak that the seminal fluid was emitted involuntarily. The slightest irritation caused an imperfect erection, immediately followed by an emission of semen,[15] which weakened him daily. The spasm, which he felt previously only on the consummation of the act, and which terminated with it, had become habitual; this often attacked him without any apparent cause, and so violently, that during the whole paroxysm, which sometimes continued fifteen hours, and never less than eight, he experienced in the posterior part of the neck, such severe pain, that he groaned, and it was impossible for him to swallow. His voice became harsh, but I did not discover it to be more so during the paroxysm. He lost all his strength, was obliged to give up his business, became fit for nothing, and was without medical aid for several months; the little of memory which remained and which soon disappeared, served only to increase his misery by recalling to mind the cause of his misfortune. I heard of his situation and went to see him; I found him more like a corpse than a living being, lying on the bed, his body dry, emaciated, pale, dirty, exhaling a disagreeable odor, and almost motionless. A pale bloody discharge issued from his nose; he foamed at his mouth, was affected with diarrhea and voided his fæces involuntarily; there was a constant discharge of seminal fluid; his eyes were watery, dim, and fixed; his pulse extremely small and frequent; respiration difficult, emaciation extreme, except in the feet which began to be edematous[16]. The mind was no less affected, his memory was gone; he was incapable of reading, without anxiety of any kind, with no sensation except that of pain which returned with every paroxysm, that occurred at least as often as once in three clays. It is difficult to form an idea of the horrid appearance of this person who was sunk far beneath the brute, and who could hardly be recognized as a human being. I soon was able, by the aid of tonics, to remove the violent spasmodic fits which recalled his sensibility by pain; satisfied with having relieved him in this respect, I discontinued remedies which could no longer be of service. He died some weeks after; the whole body edematous.

All those addicted to this odious and criminal practice are not diseased so much, as was this young man; but all are more or less affected. The frequency of the practice, the variety of temperaments, and several other circumstances, cause considerable differences. The symptoms, most frequently are: 1. A functional derangement of the stomach, apparent in some, by the loss of appetite, or by its irregularities; in others by acute pains, particularly during digestion, and by constant vomitings which resist all remedies while this practice is continued. 2. A weakness in the respiratory organs, often attended with a dry cough, generally with a hoarse, weak voice, and hurried respiration after much exertion. 3. A very great relaxation of the nervous system.

It does not require much knowledge of the physical relations existing in the animal economy, to perceive that these three causes may produce all the diseases of debility, and do produce them every day. The first symptoms which occur in those addicted to this practice are, beside those already enumerated, a great loss of strength, extreme paleness, sometimes a slight but permanent yellowness; frequently pimples, which disappear, and are as constantly replaced by others—they show themselves in every part of the face, but particularly on the forehead, temples, and near the nose; considerable emaciation, an astonishing sensibility to the changes in the weather, feebleness of sight, and a great prostration of all the mental faculties, particularly of the memory. "I am confident," says a patient who writes me, "that this pernicious practice has diminished the powers of my mind, particularly of the memory." I shall take the liberty to insert here extracts from several letters, which united will form a complete description of the physical disorders produced by masturbation, and which I did not use in the first edition because it was written in Latin. "I had the misfortune, like many other young men, to be addicted to this habit, so destructive both to the body and mind. Age, instructed by reason, restrained for some time, this criminal indulgence, but it was too late. The extraordinary nervous sensibility and the symptoms it occasions are constantly attended by a feebleness, malaise, weariness and distress. There is a constant discharge of semen; the countenance is cadaverous, pale and leaden. My very great debility renders the performance of every motion difficult, that of my legs is often so great, that I can scarcely stand erect, and I fear to leave my chamber. Digestion is so imperfect, that the food passes the bowels unchanged, three or four hours after it has been taken into the stomach. I am oppressed with phlegm, the presence of which causes pain, and the expectoration, exhaustion. This is a brief history of my miseries which are increased by the painful reflection, that each day brings with it an increase of all my woes. Nor do I believe that any human creature ever suffered more. Without a special interposition of Divine Providence, I cannot support so painful an existence." I read with astonishment in the letter of another patient, these words of shocking import, and which brought to mind those mentioned in *Onania*. "Were I not restrained by *sentiments of religion*, I should ere this have put an end to my existence, which is the more insupportable, as it is caused by myself."[17] In fact, there is no state so hard to be borne, as that of anguish of mind; pain is nothing in comparison to it, and when combined with numerous diseases of the body, it is not astonishing that such patients should desire death as their greatest good, and regard life as an evil; if we can call a state so wretched life.

> Vivere quum nequeam, sit mihi posse mori;
> Dulce mori miseris, sed mors optata recidit.
>
> —*M.*

The following description is shorter and less affecting. "I had the misfortune in the early part of my childhood, I believe between eight and ten years of age, to contract this infamous practice which soon ruined my constitution. My nerves are now very weak, my hands are powerless; they tremble and sweat continually. I have violent pains in the stomach, legs, arms, sometimes in the loins and chest; I have a frequent cough; my eyes are weak and glassy; my appetite is voracious, yet my countenance grows worse every day."

The success of remedies in this case, will be seen in the section on the treatment. The details of the cure of the first will not be given on account of their length.

"Nature," writes a third, "opens my eyes to the cause of the languor with which I am perpetually troubled, and to the dangers which threaten me. The vesicles which form on the penis, and the weakness during the act of pollution convince me that it depends on this cause."

I might add here a great number of cases of patients, who have consulted me since the second edition of this work, but these would be useless repetitions; I shall therefore mention only one or two of the most recent.

A man who is in the meridian of life, wrote me a few days as follows: "I contracted the criminal practice of self-pollution when very young, which has ruined my health; I was affected with vertigo, which made me fear apoplexy, and for which I was bled; it was soon perceived that this was wrong. My chest is contracted and my respiration consequently impeded; I have frequent pains in my stomach, and in almost every part of the body; during the day I am sleepy and restless, in the night my sleep is disturbed, and does not refresh me; I often have itchings; my eyes are weak and painful; my countenance is of a sallow paleness; my taste is depraved," etc.

"I cannot walk," writes a second, "two hundred paces without resting myself; my feebleness is extreme; I have constant pains in every part of the body, but particularly in the shoulders and chest; my appetite is good, but this is a misfortune, since whatever is eaten causes pains in the stomach and is vomited up; if I read a page or two my eyes are filled with tears and become painful; I often sigh involuntarily. *Filo xylino flaccidus veretrum, omnisque erectionis impotens, semen quidem, manu sollicitatum, effluere finit, nequa quam vero ejaculat; adeo cæterum imminutum et retractum ut oculi de se xu vix judicaret possint.*"

A third who became addicted to the same practice at the age of twelve years, was affected more in his mental faculties, than in his bodily health. "My enthusiasm is sensibly diminished; my perceptions are very dull; the fire of imagination much less vivid; every passing event appears to me like a dream; I have less power of conception, and less presence of mind; in a word I feel as if I am wasting away, although my sleep, appetite, and countenance are good."

Hypochondriasis is not unfrequent; and if those patients who labor under it give themselves up to this practice, it becomes the most prominent of the symptoms of the disease, and renders it incurable. I have seen great anxiety, restlessness, and frightful agitations, produced by the combined action of these two causes; and I have often observed, that in those hypocondriacs subject to attacks of delirium, the paroxysm was always hastened by masturbation. The cerebrum enfeebled by this double cause loses successively all its faculties, and the patients become imbecile except during attacks of phrenzy. In the *Mémoires des curieux de la nature* is mentioned the case of a man affected with melancholy, who, according to the advice of Horace, sought to drown his sorrows with wine, but being addicted to another kind of excess, became attacked soon after his second marriage with so violent a delirium, that it was necessary to chain him.

Jakin has given in his commentaries on Rhazes[18], the history of a melancholic man who, from excesses of the same kind, became affected with consumption attended with mania of which he soon died.

We know that paroxysms of epilepsy, when accompanied by an emission of seminal fluid, leave the patient more exhausted, and more confused, than in ordinary cases. Coition is an exciting cause of these fits, in those who are subject to them; and Van Swieten attributes the great exhaustion of the patients to this cause if the attacks be frequent. Didier knew a merchant of Montpelier, who never had connection of this kind without having soon after a fit of epilepsy.

Galen relates a similar case, and Henry Van Heers testifies to the same thing: this is corroborated by my own observation. Van Swieten knew an epileptic person who was attacked with a fit the night he was married. Hoffman knew a very lecherous female who generally had a fit of epilepsy after each act of venery. I will insert here Boerhaave's remarks, in his *treatise on the diseases of the nerves*, that in the *ardeur vénérienne* all the nerves are affected, and sometimes so much as to prove fatal. He relates the case of a female who fell into a very long syncope[19], after every act of coition, and that of a man who died in the first act of this kind, the force of the spasms suddenly produced a complete paralysis, and I find in Sauvages' excellent work on medicine, the very singular and perhaps unique instance of a man who, in the middle of the act, was seized with a spasm which rendered his whole body stiff, (and which continued for twelve years,) with loss of sensation and consciousness. "Ita ut illum præ oneris impotentia, in alteram lecti partem excutere cogeretur uxor, et evacuatio spermatis lenta flaccidoque veretro demum succedebat remittente corporis rigiditate." I have known several analogous facts: Haller mentions a great number, in his remarks on the *Institutes of Boerhaave*, and we find several by other observers.

We have seen above that masturbation produces epilepsy, and this happens more frequently perhaps than is generally supposed; is it astonishing that it brings on these fits, as we have seen several times, in those who are subject to them? Is it surprising that it renders this disease incurable?

This complete rigidity of the whole body mentioned by Boerhaave is one of the rarest symptoms; we had never seen it but once, when the last edition of this work was printed, but in the most perfect degree. The disease commenced by a stiffness in the neck and spine, and attacked all the limbs in succession. I saw this young man some time before death; the only position he could have was on his back, in bed; he could neither move his hands nor feet; he could take no nourishment but what was put into his mouth by others: he lived some weeks in this miserable state, and died or rather sunk away almost without suffering.

I have since seen another terrible case of this total and fatal rigidity. I was requested to visit in the country a man, forty years old, who had been very strong and robust, but who had indulged excessively in sexual commerce and in wine, and who had been often engaged in athletic exercises. He began to be affected, a few months since, by a weakness in his legs, which made him totter in his walk as if drank, he sometimes fell when walking on a plane; he could not descend the stairs without much difficulty, and hardly dared to leave his apartment. His hands trembled very much. He wrote with very great difficulty and very badly, but he dictated with ease although his speech which had never been very fluent, began to be less so. His memory was still good and the only ground for suspecting a lesion in his mind was the want of attention at the *jeu de dames*[20] and the change of countenance; his appetite was good and he slept well, but it was difficult for him to turn in bed.

It occurred to me that his gallantries and a too free use of wine, were the first causes of the disease, and that his athletic excercises in which he had been frequently engaged, were the origin of the particular affection of the muscles. The season was not favorable for the use of remedies, but it was necessary to attempt to arrest the progress of the disease. I advised frictions of the whole body with flannels, and some tonics; I directed the doses to be increased, and to add also the use of the cold bath at the commencement of summer. In a few weeks, the trembling of the hands seemed to be a little diminished. A consultation was had in the month of April; the disease was attributed to his having written some months, two years since, in a chamber recently plastered. Warm baths, oily frictions with diaphoretic and antispasmodic powders were employed without benefit. In the month of June, in a second consultation, he was advised to visit the medicinal spring of Leuk in Valais; on his return the trembling and stiffness had increased. From this time

(Sept. 1760, to Jan. 1764), I saw him but three or four times. In 1762, he procured from Frankfort the remedies mentioned in the English treatise, *Onania*, which were of no use. He consulted a foreign physician the last year with as little success. The disease has slowly but daily progressed; and for several months before death his legs were too weak to support the weight of his body; he could not move his hands nor arms without help; his speech was so embarrassed and his voice so feeble, that it was difficult to understand him; the extensor muscles of the head allowed it to fall continually on the chest; he had constant pain in the loins; his sleep and appetite was sensibly diminished; during the last few months of his life, there was much difficulty in swallowing; after Christmas there came on an irregular fever, and his eyes were singularly dim; when I saw him in the month of January he passed the whole day and most of the night reclining on a sofa with his feet in a chair, with a domestic constantly in attendance near him in order to change his position, raise his head to feed him, and to listen attentively to all he said. As he approached the period of his dissolution he was obliged to articulate letter by letter which was written down as it was pronounced. Seeing that I gave him no encouragement as I only employed some palliatives for his fever and oppression, and actuated by a desire of living, he sent one of his friends to tell me the cause to which he attributed all these symptoms, viz. *masturbation*; that he commenced this infamous practice several years since, had continued it as long as possible, and that he had perceived his difficulties increase in proportion to his indulgence in it. He confirmed this statement a few days afterward and it was this which induced him to use the remedies recommended in *Onania*.

Excesses in the gratification of sexual desires not only cause the diseases of langour, but sometimes acute diseases and they always produce irregularities in those affections which depend on other causes, and very readily render them malignant when the energies of nature are in fault.

Hippocrates has left us in his history of epidemic diseases, the case of a young man who after excesses with women and wine, was attacked with a fever, accompanied with symptoms the most violent and irregular, which finally proved fatal.

Hoffman's remarks on this subject deserve to be noticed. After speaking of the dangers of sexual gratifications in diseased subjects, he examines those of persons who have fever while thus indulging themselves, and he begins by mentioning a case given by Fabricius, of Hilden who says, that a man, having had connection with a female the tenth day from an attack of pleuritus[21] which had terminated on the seventh by perspiration, was seized with an ardent fever, and considerable tremor, and died on the thirteenth. He then mentions the history of a man, fifty years old, gouty and addicted to the same vices as mentioned in the above case of Hippocrates, who, while in the early part of his convalescence from an attack of peripenumonia notha, was seized, immediately after coition, with a relapse of all the symptoms of the disease, but much more violent and dangerous than at first, with a general tremor and an excessive redness of countenance. He mentions a man who never indulged in venereal excess without the supervention of fever which continued several days. He concludes with the remarks of Bartholin who knew a person attacked the next day after marriage with acute fever, weakness of the stomach, nausea, immoderate thirst, wakefulness and restlessness. He was cured by rest and some strengthening medicines.

N. Chesneau knew two young married persons attacked, the first week of their marriage, with a violent fever and considerable redness and swelling of the face; one of them had a severe pain in the sacrum22: they both died in a few days.

Vandermonde describes a fever produced by the same cause, which was also very long and attended with the most frightful symptoms, but which terminated more favourably than the case of Hippocrates. His description is too long to insert here but we advise its perusal. We shall give the treatment hereafter. De Sauvages describes this disease under the name *fièvre ardente des épuisés*[23]; the pulse is sometimes strong and full, and sometimes weak and small, urine high colored, skin dry and hot, great thirst, nausea and wakefulness.

I knew, in 1761 and 1762, two very healthy, strong and vigorous young men who were attacked, one the day after, and the other the second night of their marriage, with a very violent fever, preceded by no chill, pulse quick and hard, wakefulness, many slight convulsive motions, very great inquietude, and dry skin; the appearance of the second was very much altered, and he was troubled with dysuria[24]. I first thought that an intemperate use of wine was in part the procuring cause of these symptoms, but I was of a different opinion in regard to the second. They were cured at the end of two days. This circumstance added to the character of the disease, leaves no doubt of the cause.

Some deplorable cases have taught me that acute diseases in those addicted to masturbation are very dangerous; their progress is generally irregular, their symptoms deceptive, their periods deranged; we find no resources in the constitution; art is obliged to do every thing; and as a perfect crisis never takes place, when the disease is subdued with much trouble, the patient remains in a state of languor, rather than of convalescence, which requires the most assiduous attention, to prevent it from assuming a chronic form; and we know, that Fonseca was aware of this danger. Some young men, says he, even when very robust, are affected after excesses with females, the same night, with an acute fever which destroys them, or they are attacked with severe diseases which are difficult to cure; for if, when the body is weakened by venereal excesses, it be attacked by acute affections there is no remedy.

A young man, not sixteen years old, became addicted to masturbation to so great a degree, that finally, instead of semen there was an emission of blood, which was followed by excessive pain and inflammation of all the genital organs. Finding me accidentally in the country, I was consulted; I ordered extremely emollient cataplasms[25] which produced the expected effect; but I have since learned that he died shortly after with small pox, and doubtless the injury done the constitution by these bad practices, contributed very much to render the disease mortal. What a warning to young men!

All those who have had occasion to treat the venereal disease, know that it is often fatal in subjects exhausted by frequent debauchery. Of this we have seen most horrid instances.

SECTION V.

CONSEQUENCES OF MASTURBATION IN FEMALES.

The preceding remarks except that of Stehelin, seem to apply principally to males; this subject would be imperfectly treated, did we not warn females, that, in pursuing the same course, they will be exposed to the same dangers; that it has, more than once, produced all the evils we have mentioned, and that every day some of those addicted to this practice perish its miserable victims. The English treatise *Onania*, is filled with cases which cannot be read without horror and compassion; the disease even seems to be more active in females, than in males. Besides all the symptoms we have mentioned, they are more particularly subject to attacks of hysteria, melancholy, incurable jaundice, acute pains in the stomach and back, fluor albus the acridity of which is a constant source of acute suffering, prolapsus and ulceration of the uterus and their consequences, to elongations of the clitoris and furor uterinus which deprives them both of modesty and reason, and places them on a level with the most lascivious brutes, until death terminates their career.

The countenance, that faithful mirror of the soul and body, is the first to indicate these internal derangements. The healthy appearance and the color which unite to form that air of youth, which alone can supply the place of beauty, and without which, beauty itself produces no sensation but that of cold admiration, appear first; emaciation, lividity of the countenance, and roughness of the skin, immediately follow; the eyes lose their lustre and indicate by their languor that of the whole system; the lips lose their redness, the teeth their whiteness, and finally, the development of the body is not unfrequently checked and the figure deformed.

Rachitis[26] is not a disease as Boerhaave states, which never occurs after the age of three years. It is commonly seen in young people, of both sexes, particularly among females who, after being well formed till after eight, ten and even sixteen years of age, suddenly become deformed by a curvature of the spine, and the derangement is sometimes very great. We shall not here mention the details of this disease, nor enumerate the causes which produce it. Hippocrates has mentioned two. We shall perhaps have occasion to mention in another work our information on this subject gained from several cases; but we ought to remark in this place, that among these causes, onanism stands first.

Hoffman had already remarked, that young people who are addicted to the pleasures of love, before their growth is terminated, become thin and emaciated; and we know that a cause which can prevent the growth, can also disturb its arrangement and produce those irregularities in its progress, which contribute to the disease of which we are speaking.

A symptom, common to the two sexes, and which we shall mention in this article, because it is more common in females, is the indifference produced by this vice for the lawful pleasures of marriage even when the powers and desires are not exhausted; an indifference which not only leads to celibacy, but often follows them to the marriage-bed. A woman, mentioned by Dr. Bekkers, asserts that this vice has produced such an effect on her senses, that she has no inclination for lawful intercourse. I know a man who instructed in this by his preceptor, had the same disgust at the commencement of marriage ; and the anguish of this situation added to exhaustion, made him very melancholy; he was however cured by tonics and nervines[27].

Before proceeding farther, let me invite mothers and fathers to reflect on the cause of the unhappiness of this last patient, and there are more than one in the same situation; if perhaps deceived on this subject in the choice of those to whom is entrusted the important charge of forming the mind and affections of young men, what ought they not to fear, both from those who being destined to develop their bodily capabilities, are examined less strictly in regard to their morals, and from the domestics who are often employed without ascertaining whether they have any? The child mentioned by Rast, of Montpelier, was instructed in this vice by a servant girl; the English collection is full of such instances, and we know of too many young plants which have been lost by the gardener to whom the care of their cultivation was committed. In this kind of cultivation there are gardeners of both sexes. What remedies are there for these evils? It is not for me to answer and I shall be brief. Be very careful in choosing a preceptor and watch over him and his pupil with that vigilance by which an enlightened and attentive father discovers what is happening in the most obscure parts of his house:

> Docuit enim fabula dominium videre plurimum in rebus suis.
> —Plæd.

Never leave young pupils alone with tutors suspected, and prohibit all intercourse with domestics.

A short time since, a girl, eighteen years of age, who had enjoyed very good health, became very weak, her strength daily diminished, she was constantly affected with drowsiness during the day and wakefulness through the night; her appetite failed and her whole body became edematous. She consulted a skillful surgeon who, after learning there was no derangement in the menses[28], suspected *onanism.* The effect produced by his first question, confirmed his suspicion which was rendered certain by the confession of the patient: he advised her of the danger of this practice; in a short time the disease was arrested by remedies, and the patient discovered some amendment.

Beside *masturbation* or *manustrapation*, there is the *souillure clitoridienne* the origin of which must be ascribed to the second *Sappho.*

> Lesbides, infamem quae me fecistis, amatæ;

And which, too common among the females of Rome, at that period when all morals were degraded, was more than once the object of the epigrams and satires of the age;

Leonum ancillas posita Laufella corona
Provocat, et tollit pendentis praemia coxæ.
Ipsa Medullina frictum trissantis adorat.
Palmam inter dominas virtus natalibus æquat.[29]

Nature, in her freaks, has given some females a partial resemblance to males, whom careless observers have called *hermaphrodites.*

The preternatural length of the part which is very small, and on which Tronchin has written a learned desertation, causes the phenomenon, and the hateful abuse of it, the evil. Vain perhaps of this kind of resemblance, some of these imperfect females have attempted to perform the functions of the male.[30]

The danger in this is no less, than in other excesses; the consequences are frightful. All these abuses produce exhaustion, languor, pains and death. This last kind deserves more particular attention as it is common in our times, and it would be easy to find more than one *Laufella* and *Medullina*[31], who like these Romans, esteem the gifts of nature so much as to think to banish the arbitrary differences she has imposed. Some females have been known to love others of their sex with as much ardor as the most passionate men, and even to be jealous of those who seem to entertain for them sentiments of affection.

It is time to finish such sad details; I am weary of describing the turpitude and misery of humanity. We shall give no more cases here; those which remain will be found in their proper places; and we pass to the examination of causes, after remarking generally, that those young persons who are born with feeble constitutions have much more to fear, than those who are more vigorous. No one escapes chastisement, but it is not equally severe upon all. Those especially who are affected with hereditary diseases, as gout, calculus, phthisis, hæmoptisis, epilepsy and tabes dorsalis; all these unfortunate persons should be intimately persuaded that every act of this kind affects their constitutions very much, suddenly hastens the ills they dread, renders their attacks much more serious and will bring upon them in the bloom of life all the infirmities of old age.

Tartareas vivum constat inire vias.

ARTICLE II.

CAUSES.

SECTION VI.

IMPORTANCE OF THE SEMEN.

How does a profuse evacuation of semen cause all the symptoms we have enumerated? This is what we are now to examine. The causes may be reduced to two, the loss of this fluid and the circumstances which attend its emission. The anatomical description of the organs which secrete it, the more or less probable conjectures on the manner in which its secretion takes place, and remarks on its sensible qualities, would be out of place here. We here intend only to prove its utility by the testimonies of the most respectable physicians; we have already mentioned some of them and determined its effects upon the body. The following section will be appropriated to the examination of the effects produced by the circumstances attending emission.

Hippocrates thought it was secreted from the whole body but particularly from the head. He observes that the semen of the male comes from all the humors of the body and is the most important part of them. This is proved by the feebleness of those who lose it by coition to any extent however slight. Veins and nerves proceed from all parts of the body to the genital organs; when these are filled and warmed they communicate a pleasurerable sensation to the whole body; the humors become as it were fomented, by which all that is valuable and balsamic is separated from the rest, and is carried by the spinal marrow to the genital organs. Galen adopts this opinion. "This humor" he remarks, "is only the most subtle parts of all of them; it has veins and nerves which go from all parts of the body to the testicles. In emissions of semen," he remarks in another place, "we lose at the same time the vital spirit; it is not therefore surprising that too frequent coition enervates, since it deprives the body of its purest parts."

The same author has mentioned in his *History of Philosophy*, the opinions of the different ancient philosophers on this subject, which we shall quote here. Aristotle, whose writings on medicine will be valued as long as observations the most meritorious and difficult, terms it the most perfect part of the food, which has the power of reproducing bodies similar to those by which it is formed. Pythagoras calls it the *flower* of the purest blood. Alcmæon, his pupil, a distinguished physician, one of the first to appreciate the importance of dissecting animals, and who, among the pagan philosophers, seems to have had the most correct notions in regard to the soul; considered it, a *portion* of the *cerebrum*; and only two or three years since, a celebrated physician adopted and amplified this system; he points out the passages through which the brain passes to the testes which he regards as ganglions and not as glands, and it is by the dissipation of the brain, that he explains the phenomena of venereal exhaustion.

Plato considers this fluid as coming from the *spinal marrow*. Democritus has the same opinion as Hippocrates and Galen. Epicurus, that respectable author, who knew better than any one else that man's happiness depends on his pleasures, but who at the same time has fixed them by rules not disavowed by the Christian, yet his doctrines have been so perverted and abused by stoics, that he is considered by those who know him only through this medium, a debauchee whom Fenelon asserts to have been a man of exemplary continence, and whose manners were always moral, and I shall add, whose principles are censured severely by those pretended modern sectarians who know him only by name, and abuse him for authorizing practices which he detested, and those who love the truth ought not to suffer his memory to be dishonored, if it could be by such persons, Epicurus, I say, regarded the semen as a *part* of the *soul* and *body* and prescribed rules for carefully preserving it.

Although several of these opinions differ in some measure, yet all prove the value of this fluid.

It has been asked, Is it analogous to any other humor? Is it the same as that termed *animal spirits*, which, passing through the nerves, concurs in all the least important functions of the system, and the depravity of which produces an infinity of evils so frequent and trivial? To answer these questions positively, we must know intimately the nature of these two fluids. We are far from this degree of knowledge, and can only mention ingenious and probable conjectures.

"One easily understands," says Hoffman, "why there is so intimate a connection between the brain and the testicles, since these two organs separate from the blood the most subtle and exquisite lymph which is destined to give power and motion to parts, and even to fulfill the functions of the soul. The too great discharge of these fluids must inevitably destroy the powers of the mind and body." "The seminal fluid," he adds in another place, "is distributed like the animal spirits, separated by the brain, in all the nerves of the body: it seems to be of the same nature, hence the more it is dissipated, the less it is separated from the spirits." Gorter has the same idea. "The semen is the most perfect and the most important of the animal fluids, that which results from all the digestions; its intimate relations with the animal spirits proves that, like them, it comes from the most perfect humors." In a word, it seems from these proofs and from numerous others which it would be tedious to cite, that it is an extremely important secretion, called the *huile essentielle*[32], *quintessence* of the animal fluids, or more exactly, the *rectified spirit*, the dissipation of which leaves the other humors feeble.

However important this semen may be, since it is separated from the fluids, and is deposited in its reservoirs, of what use is it to the body? It is admitted that a too profuse evacuation of the fluids which actually circulate in the vessels and thus even supply nutrition, as the blood, the serum, the lymph, etc., should weaken; but it is more difficult to understand how a fluid, which does not circulate and which is insulated, can produce the effect. I answer, first, that similar instances which are too frequent not to be generally known, should prevent this objection. Every one has seen that an evacuation of milk (to confine ourselves to this), although moderate and not very long, weakens to such a degree that the effects sometimes continue during the rest of life, as in a nurse whose health is not vigorous, and the most robust after a certain time. The reason of it is evident: in emptying the reservoirs destined to receive the fluids, too often, in accordance with that necessity which is imposed by the laws of the system, they flow there more abundantly this secretion becomes excessive; all the others suffer, especially nutrition, which is only a species of secretion. The animal languishes and becomes weak. But in the second place we can explain that of the semen in a way in which we cannot that of the milk; the milk is simply a nutritious fluid, the too great secretion of which can injure only by diminishing too much its quantity in the circulating fluids: the semen is an active liquor, the presence of which is necessary for the performance of the functions of the organs which cease when it is discharged; the too frequent emissions of semen injure them in two ways. We will explain: some humors, as perspiration, leave the body as soon as separated from the other fluids, and are expelled from the vessels of circulation. There are others, as the urine, which when secreted is retained for a certain time in reservoirs for this purpose and until their quantity irritates them mechanically to contract and expel them. A third kind is separated and retained, like the second, in reservoirs not to be entirely evacuated, but to be perfected and thus become fit for new functions when they again enter the mass of circulating fluids. Such among others is the semen. It is secreted by the testicles thence passes through rather a long canal (the *epididymis* and *vas deferens*) into the vesiculæ seminales and is constantly taken up again by absorbent vessels and returned into the mass of circulating fluids. This fact is demonstrated by sufficient proofs, one of which will here suffice. In a healthy man the semen is constantly secreted in the testicles; it proceeds from thence into the receptacles which are very limited and which perhaps cannot contain what is secreted in one day; there are however some very continent men who have no emission of semen for whole years. What then becomes of it, if it be not returned to the circulation? This return is much facilitated by the structure of the organs which serve to secrete, to carry and to preserve it. The veins are here much larger than the arteries, and in a proportion greater than is found in any other part.33 It is probable that this absorption does not take place solely in the *vesiculæ seminales*, but also in the testicles, in the *epididymi*, which are a kind of first receptacles adhering to them, and in the *vas deferens*, through which the semen passes from these organs to the *vesiculæ seminales.*

Galen knew that the fluids were enriched by the retained semen, although he was ignorant of the manner. "All is full of it," said he, "in those who have no sexual intercourse, and we find none in those, who frequently indulge in it." He then attempts to discover, how a small quantity of this fluid can give so much energy to the body, and finally concludes, "that it is by its *exquisite virtue*, and that it thus communicates its influence very promptly to all parts of the body." He then proves, by several instances, that a trivial cause, often produces great effects, and thus concludes, "Is it then surprising, that the testicles supply a fluid capable of imparting new strength to the body? The cerebrum is truly the cause of sensation, and motion, and the heart of pulsation in the arteries." I shall conclude this section by giving the opinion of one of the greatest men of the age, in respect to the semen. "The semen is retained in the vesiculæ seminales until it is used, or expended by nocturnal emissions. During all this time, the quantity existing there excites the sexual desires of the animal; but the greatest part, the most volatile, the most odorous, that which has the most power, is resumed by the blood, and produces on entering it, remarkable changes, the hairs, and the beard; it alters the voice and the manners, for age does not produce these changes in animals; they are caused by the semen alone, as they never occur in eunuchs."

How does the semen produce these effects? This is one of the problems, which as yet cannot be solved. Probably, however, this fluid is a *stimulus* which irritates the parts with which it comes in contact; its strong odor and its evident irritation upon the genital organs leaves no doubt on this point, and it is easily understood, that these acrid particles may become constantly absorbed and mixed with the fluids, slightly but uninterruptedly stimulating the vessels to contract more forcibly; their action on the fluids is more powerful; the circulation is quickened and nutrition becomes more perfect; when this supply is deficient, several functions are never developed, as is the case in eunuchs.

Here a question naturally arises, Why do not eunuchs experience the same bad effects as those who are exhausted by venereal debauchery? We shall not answer this question until we come to the end of the next section.

SECTION VII.

EXAMINATION OF THE CIRCUMSTANCES WHICH ACCOMPANY EMISSIONS.

There are several evacuations which occur imperceptibly; all the others take place in a state of perfect health, so easily that they have no influence on the rest of the system; the most trifling action, in the organ which contains the matter to be excreted, produces its expulsion. It is not so in the evacuation of the semen. It is nothing less than a general shock, a convulsion of all the parts, an increase of the rapidity of the movements of all the fluids, to displace and expel it. Is it too great presumption to say, we must regard this necessary concurrence of the whole system, at the moment of its evacuation, as a rational proof of its influence on the body? "Coition," says Democritus, "is a kind of epilepsy." "It is," says Haller, "an action very violent, similar to a convulsion, and which of itself astonishingly weakens and affects the whole nervous system." We have seen in the cases, which I have reported above, and in those which I have quoted, emissions accompanied by convulsions, a species of epilepsy; and the same observation furnishes evident proofs of the influence, which these violent actions have on the health of the unfortunate individual in whom they occur. The promptitude with which the weakness follows the act, appears to many people, and with reason, a proof that this cannot be occasioned by merely a loss of semen; but the debility of all those affected with convulsive diseases, proves that the weakness is produced by the spasm; that which follows fits of epilepsy is sometimes excessive.

We must attribute to the spasm alone, the effect produced by coition in an a man of a Swiss village, mentioned by F. Platerus, who, being remarried when old, anxious to consummate his nuptials, was affected with a suffocation so violent, that he was obliged to desist. The same thing occurred every time he repeated the attempt. He consulted a crowd of quacks; one assured him, after he had procured and taken several medicines, that he was no more in danger. He hazarded a new attempt on this advice: his success was the same as before; but full of confidence, he persevered, and died in the act, in the arms of his wife.

The violent palpitations, which sometimes accompany coition are also a convulsive symptom. Hippocrates speaks of a young man, in whom excesses in wine, and sexual commerce, had produced, among other symptoms constant palpitations;[35] and Dolaeus, has seen one seized in the act, with a palpitation so violent, that he would have been suffocated, had he persisted. We find in Hoffman other similar facts.

The case of the child cited above is besides a proof of the prostrating influence of convulsions, which did not escape the sagacity of Rast, since at this age, he was able to evacuate only a little of the secretion of the prostate gland, and not genuine semen.

These remarks have been made by most of the best authors who have written on this subject. Galen has made this observation. "Voluptuousness," says he, "weakens the vital powers." Fleming, has not omitted this cause in his fine poem on the diseases of the nerves:

> Quin etiam nervos frangit quæcunque voluptas.

Sanctorius affirms positively that the convulsions weaken more than the emissions of semen; and it is very strange that Gotter, his commentator should have sought to prove the contrary. The reason which he gives for this difference of opinion, that these motions do not weaken more than other movements, because they are not convulsive, will not persuade any one.

An example, even were he able to adduce one, would not make it a law. Listel, Noguez, and Quincy who had commented on the same work before him, did not think with him, for they attributed one part of the danger to the feebleness produced by the convulsions. Coition, says Noguez, is a convulsion; it disposes the nerves to spasmodic actions, which are excited by the slightest cause.

J. B, Borelli, one of the earliest physiologists, did not think with Gotter; he is positive on this point: "this act is accompanied by a kind of convulsive action, which powerfully affects the brain and nerves."

Senac attributes positively to the nerves the feebleness which follows coition. The most probable cause of syncope, which ensues, when an abscess opens within the abdomen is, says he, "the action of the nerves which then come into play." This is confirmed by the faintness or syncope which follows the emission of semen; for we must impute this faintness to the nerves. Lewis attributes it more to this cause than to the other.

When convulsions occur, the nervous system is in a state of excitement, or more properly in a degree of extraordinary action, which is necessarily followed by an extreme relaxation. Whenever the action of an organ is over-excited, depression succeeds; hence its functions are necessarily deranged, and as the nerves have an influence on all, every part is deranged when they are enfeebled.

One reason which contributes also to the debility of the nervous system, is the increased quantity of blood in the brain, during coition, which has been perfectly demonstrated and has several times produced apoplexy: several such instances have been reported; and Hoffman states that a soldier, much addicted to this practice, finally died in the act: the cerebrum was found full of blood. This increase of blood in the brain, explains why these excesses produce mania. As this quantity of blood oppresses the nerves, it weakens: they are more susceptible of impressions and hence then debility.

When we reflect on the effects of these two causes, the emission of the semen, and the convulsive motions, the disorders arising from them are easily explained. They may be arranged in three classes: disorder of the digestive organs, debility of the brain and nervous system, and derangement of the perspiration. Every chronic disease can be produced by these three causes.

The debility caused by these excesses, deranges the functions of all the organs, says one of the best authors who has written on dietetics; digestion, perspiration, and the other evacuations, do not take place in their usual healthy manner; hence the strength, the memory, and even the understanding, are evidently diminished; the sight is obscured; diseases of the nerves and all kinds of gouty and rheumatic pains, and astonishing weakness in the back, debility in the genital organs, bloody urine, deranged appetite, headache, and numerous other diseases ensue: in a word, nothing shortens life so much as the abuse of sexual pleasures.

1. The stomach is the part first affected by any of the causes of debility, because its functions require the greatest perfection in the organ. Most of the others are as much passive as active; the stomach is almost entirely active; when its strength is diminished, its functions are also deranged; this fact, added to the succession and variety of first and often pernicious effects produced on the food in this viscus, account for the frequency and stubbornness of its diseases. Of all parts of the body it is one of those which receive the greatest number of nerves, and in which consequently is received the greatest amount of nervous influence. Whatever then weakens the action of the one, diminishes the quantity or the quality of the other, must then effect the power of this viscus more than any other; this is the case in excesses in venery. Its functions are so important that when they are not well performed, all others are affected.

> "Hujus enim validus firmat tenor omnia membra;
> At contra ejusdem frangunjur cuncta dolore."

When digestion is imperfect, the fluids become so crude that they are unfit for the uses they are destined to perform, particularly for nutrition on which the re-establishment of the strength depends. In order to be convinced of the general influence of the stomach over the other functions, it is only necessary to observe a person affected with dyspepsia[35]. In a short time he becomes weak, the organs are deranged, the senses are blunted, the faculties of the mind are exercised imperfectly, the memory, and particularly the imagination, seem dull; in short nothing renders a man apparently more stupid than indigestion, when it becomes a disease.

A fine case reported by Payva, a Portuguese physician resident at Rome, throws great light on the debility produced in the stomach by excesses of this kind.

"When the venereal desires" says he, "felt in young men, arrive to the greatest degree, they experience a kind of agreeable sensation at the pit of the stomach; but if they satisfy this inclination with too much impetuosity and beyond their strength, they have an extremely disagreeable sensation in the same place, which they cannot describe, and they pay dearly for this indulgence by debility, marasmus[36], etc. into which they fall."[37]

Aretæus was aware of this; and Boerhaave expresses himself like Payva; he adds, this painful sensation disappears as they resume their strength; in another place he confirms the same thing, adding a very useful practical rule, that when epilepsy is the consequence of indulgence in venery, we should endeavour to strengthen the nerves of the stomach.

2. The feebleness of the nervous system, which disposes to all paralytic and spasmodic affections, is produced as we have already mentioned by the convulsive actions which attend emissions: and in the second place by indigestion: when this is the case the nerves are the parts most affected, inasmuch as the preparation of the fluids which goes to them is the highest function of digestion, of that which is supposed to be the most perfect; when it is deranged, this is the most altered of any of the animal fluids, and in which crudity has the most effect. Finally, this debility is increased by the evacuation of a fluid analogous to the animal spirits, and on account of this analogy it cannot be evacuated without diminishing the energies of the nervous system, and we are not prevented from attributing this consequence to the animal spirits, by the modest doubts of some great men who dare affirm only what falls under their own observation, or by the doubts of more systematic physiologists. Besides, independent of the injury resulting from this evacuation in regard to the quantity of animal spirits with which it may be blended, it is injurious, as it deprives the vessels of the slight stimulus which is produced by the absorbed semen, which contributes so much to the perfection of the fluids, and which would otherwise be imperfect.

The relation between the diseases of the stomach, and those of the nerves, is reciprocal. The former produce the latter, and when these are once formed, they very much increase them. Were this not proved by daily observation, the anatomical inspection of the stomach would be sufficient to support it. The number of its nerves demonstrates how necessary they are for the performance of its functions, and how easily they may be deranged when they are not in health.

3. Finally, the perspiration goes on less perfectly. Sanctorius has even determined the quantity which is lost by it: and this evacuation, the most considerable of all, when suppressed must necessarily result in a crowd of different symptoms.

It is easy to comprehend that all diseases may be produced by these three causes. I shall not enter into an explanation of all the particular symptoms; to detail them would be to extend this work too much, and would interest physicians alone: Gotter's work on perspiration may be consulted.

Clifton Wintringham has given a very good description of the dangers arising from derangements of this evacuation in persons affected with gout, and his explanation deserves to be read.

Feu Gunzius, an eminent physician in the flower of his age, has given a very ingenious mechanical explanation of the symptoms in respect to respiration; he mentions under this head a man who was affected with constant cough, a symptom which I saw in a young man who died a victim to onanism. He came to Montpelier to pursue his studies; his excesses in this practice produced phthisis, and I remember his cough was so loud and hard as to incommode his neighbors.

He was frequently bled, doubtless to relieve his sufferings. A consultation of physicians was called; they prescribed turtle soup and a return home, as he was a native of Dauphiny, and promised him a perfect cure. He died two hours afterwards.

It is more difficult, or rather we are unable, to understand why the faculties of the mind are so much enfeebled. The solution of this problem depends upon what we do not understand, the reciprocal action of the body and mind upon each other and we must therefore observe the phenomena. We are ignorant both of the nature of the mind and that of the body: but we know in man the two are intimately united, and that all the changes in the one are felt in the other; a slight alteration in the circulation, in the viscidity of the blood, in the quantity or in the quality of the food, as a cup of coffee instead of a little wine, in the length or the tranquility of sleep, an excess or diminution of the dejections, or of perspiration, affects our views and opinions of objects; the changes in the functions of the system alter our thoughts and sentiments and inspire in their turn new notions of virtues and vices: so true are the remarks of the first modern satirist, Regnier, that they are inserted.

> Tout, suivant l'intellect, change d'ordre et de rang:
> Ainsi c'est la nature et l'humeur des personnes,
> Et non la qualité qui rend les choses bonnes.
> C'est un mal bien etrange au cerveau des humains.

The following is a correct description of this intimate unioa drawn by Lucretius.

—Gigni pariter cum corpore, et una
Crescere sentimus, pariturque senescere mentem.
Nam velut infirmo pueri teneroque vagantu
Corpore, sic animi sequitur sententia tenuis.
Inde ubi robustis adolevit viribus ætas,
Consilium quoque majus, et auctior est animi vis:
Post ubi jam validis quassatum est viribus ævi
Corpus, et obtusis ceciderunt viribus artus;
Claudicat ingenium, delirat linguaque, mensque.
Omnia deficiunt, atque uno tempore desunt:
Quin etiam morbis in corporis avius errat.
Sæpe animus, dementit enim deliraque fatur.

Observation also teaches that of all the diseases there is no one which affects the mind so soon as that of the nervous system; those epileptic persons who, after some years, become imbecile, furnish a sad proof of this, which removes our astonishment that those addicted to this habit are always slightly epileptic, and that imbecility of the mental faculties follows as a consequence.

Weakness of the brain and nervous system is naturally followed by that of the senses. Sanctorius, Hoffman, and some others have attempted to explain why the sight suffers more particularly, but their reasons although correct, do not seem to us sufficient. The principal reasons and those peculiar to this organ are that the number of its component parts, all of which being subject to different diseases, render it infinitely more liable to derangements. The nerves also serve here for several uses, and are very numerous. Finally the rush of fluids to these during the act, which is indicated by the scintillations then observed in the eyes of animals, produces in the vessels first a weakness, then engorgements, which are necessarily followed with loss of sight.

It is in fact easy to answer the question proposed above, why are eunuchs in whom there is no secretion of semen not exposed to the diseases we have described?

There are two sufficient reasons, the first is they do not enjoy the benefit of the semen when it has been secreted and reabsorbed, and secondly they do not lose at all the precious part of the blood which composes it. They do not experience the changes arising from the semen, and which we have mentioned above; but they are not exposed to the evils caused by the privations of this fluid. I might, if allowed to use metaphysical expressions, distinguish the seminal fluid into semen in potentia which is the most precious part, and the semen in actu. If the first is not secreted, the system is deprived of its influence, and does not experience the changes which depend on it; but it does not enfeeble them; it is not formed and consequently is not lost; they continue in a state similar to that of infancy. When the semen is secreted and evacuated, there is a loss, a real waste. The second reason is that eunuchs suffer no spasms lo which we have attributed most of the bad consequences resulting from this abuse.

The symptoms which supervene in females, are explained like those in men. The secretion which they lose, being less valuable and less matured than the semen of the male, its loss does not enfeeble so promptly, but when they indulge in it to excess, as their nervous system is naturally weaker and more disposed to spasms, the symptoms are more violent.

Sudden excesses produce symptoms similar to those of the young man mentioned above, and we have seen a case of this kind. In 1746, a prostitute, twenty-three years of age, had connection in a single night with six Spanish dragoons near Montpelier. The next morning she was brought into the city in a dying state; she expired in the evening bathed in uterine hemorrhage which flowed in a constant stream. It would have been very interesting to have ascertained whether this hemorrhage was in consequence of a wound or depended only on a dilatation of the vessels produced by an increased action in them.

SECTION VIII.

CAUSES OF THE DANGERS PECULIAR TO MASTURBATION.

We have seen that masturbation is more pernicious than excessive intercourse with females. Those who believe in a special providence, account for it by a special ordinance of the Deity to punish this crime.[38]

Satisfied that our bodies have been subjected from their birth to laws which necessarily regulate all its functions, the diversity of which does not change the economy, except in a few instances, we wish to explain by miracles, only what ever is evidently in opposition to physical causes. This is not the case here: all can be explained very well, by the mechanism of the body and by its union with the mind. This habit of recurring to supernatural causes, has been contested by Hippocrates who, in speaking of a disease regarded by the Scythians as a special punishment from the Deity, makes this excellent remark, "it is true this disease came from God, but it comes from him only like all other diseases: they all are a consequence of the laws of nature which governs every thing."

Sanctorius in his remarks mentions a first cause of this peculiar danger; "coition," says he "in a moderate degree is useful, when it is solicited by nature, but when it is excited by the imagination it enfeebles all the faculties of the mind, and particularly the memory. The reason of this is evident. Nature in a state of health excites the desires only when the seminal vesicles are filled with the semen, which has become so thick as to render its resolution more difficult, and this indicates that its loss will not sensibly weaken the body. But such is the structure of the genital organs, that their excitation and the desires which follow, are brought into action, not only by the presence of an abundance of seminal fluid, but also by the imagination which has much influence on these parts; by engrossing the thoughts, it can excite them, and desire leads to the act which is more pernicious, because more unnecessary. It is with the organs of this system as with those of all the others which are properly brought into action only by nature. Hunger and thirst indicate the necessity for food and drink; if we take more than these sensations demand, the surplus is injurious to the body and debilitates it. The necessity of evacuating feces and urine is also marked by certain physical conditions; but the constitution of the organs may be so perverted by bad habit, that it ceases to depend on the quantity of matter to be evacuated. These wants are satisfied when there is no necessity, and this is the case with masturbators. It is the imagination, the habit, and not nature, which requires them. They deprive nature of what is necessary for her healthful operations. Finally, in consequence of this law in the animal economy, that the fluids flow more abundantly to those parts which become irritated, there is after a certain time, a continual rush to them; and the remark of Hippocrates is verified that, 'when a man has connection, the seminal veins are dilated and solicit the semen.'"

We may remark here that masturbation is particularly injurious to children before the age of puberty; happily we find but few monsters of either sex who indulge in it before this period, still the number is too great. Numerous circumstances prevent illicit intercourse with females, but a solitary debauchee is confined by no limit and restrained by no obstacle.

A second cause is the dominion it obtains over the senses, which has been well described in the English treatise, *Onania*. "This immodesty," says the author, "has no sooner subjugated the heart, than it follows the criminal every where; it takes possession of his mind in every place, in the most serious pursuits, even in those of religion; he is a prey to the most lascivious ideas which never leave him." Nothing weakens so much as this continual excitement of a mind always intent on the same thing. A person addicted to this habit, experiences the same ill effects as does the literary man who fixes his attention wholly on one subject. This part of the brain, which is then in action, makes an effort which may be compared to that of a muscle which has been powerfully and for a long time extended; this is followed either by so much motion that the play of the part cannot be arrested, nor the mind be diverted from this idea, (this is the case in those addicted to onanism); or by a perfect impotence. Finally exhausted by continual fatigue, these patients are affected with all the diseases of the brain, melancholy, catalepsy, epilepsy, imbecility, loss of sense, feebleness of the nervous system, and a multitude of other evils. It very much injures numerous young men; since even when their faculties are not exhausted, their use is perverted. Whatever be their pursuit, they succeed in nothing without a degree of attention which is impossible, on account of this destructive habit. Among those who have no business, (and of these there are too many,) there are some not fit for this; an air of distraction, embarrassment and stupidity, causes only a disagreeable feeling of laziness. We might also mention that this inability to confine the attention added to the diminution of the faculties entirely incapacitates for taking any stand in society. This sad state reduces man below the level of the brute, and justly renders him an object of contempt more than of pity.

These first two causes are necessarily attended by a third, which is the frequency of the act; the mind and body concur when once the habit is by any means powerful, to solicit this indulgence. The mind, a prey to libidinous thoughts, excites the body to lasciviousness, and if it be diverted some moments by other ideas, the acrid fluids which irritate the genital organs soon excite to abuse. How effectual would these remarks be in arresting young men, if they could foresee that here one false step causes another; that when they are almost subdued by temptation, and that in proportion as the motives of seduction increase, reason which should restrain them becomes enfeebled: they are finally plunged into an abyss of msery, from which they cannot be saved. If sometimes commencing infirmities give them strong advice, if the danger terrifies them for some moments, the fury for this vice pushes them onward and they may well exclaim.

> I know the right, and I approve it too;
> I know the wrong, and yet the wrong pursue.

The danger however is near, and the time for amendment is short.

> Canis et manes et fabula fies.
> Vive memor lethi, fugit hora; hoc quodliquoi inde est.
> —Pers. I.

While I was studying philosophy at Geneva, a time I shall ever remember, one of my schoolmates had arrived at that horrid state, that he could not abstain from this evil practice even during the time of recitation, but he was soon punished, for he died in about two years of consumption. A similar case is mentioned in the work, *Onania*. The ingenious author who has quoted from my Latin treatise in the excellent Latin journal published at Berne, mentions that a whole school sometimes strove, by this practice, to dissipate the ennui and keep themselves awake during the lectures upon scholastic metaphysics, delivered by a sleepy professor, but this seems not so much to prove what I advanced, as the horrid dissipation into which young men may fall.

The same author has recently published in a work which I cannot read, but which is considered by an excellent judge to be one of the best productions of the age the following: Some years since, it was discovered in the city, that a company of libertines, fourteen or fifteen years old, used to assemble to practice this vice, and that a whole school is still polluted by it.

The health of a young prince was gradually declining and the reason could not be ascertained. His surgeon suspected the cause, watched, and detected him in the act: he said that one of his valets had instructed him in it, and that he practiced it frequently. The habit was so strong, that the most pressing considerations forcibly stated to him could not eradicate it. The evil progressed, he lost strength daily, and was saved only by guarding him day and night for more than eight months.

A patient in one of his letters to me gives a vivid description of the difficulties to be overcome. "It is necessary to use great efforts, these are the terms for subduing a habit which is recalled to mind every instant. I blush to assure you that the sight of a female object, whatever it may be, excites in me these desires. I have no want of this help, for my mind is constantly employed in representing to me the objects of concupiscence. This passion does not excite me much; it is true I constantly remember all your advice; I combat it but even that contest wastes me. If you are able to find the means to turn aside my thoughts from these objects, I believe that my cure will soon be accomplished."

We have already seen in an extract from *Onania*, that the frequent repetition had produced furor uterinus in a female. The habit of being occupied with one idea incapacitates for others; it becomes supreme and reigns despotically: the organs constantly irritated contract a morbid tendency, which becomes a constant source of irritation independent of any external cause. Some diseases of the urinary organs, excite a continual incontinence of urine; the constant irritation of the genital organs produces a similar disease. It is not astonishing that the concurrence of these two moral and physical causes should produce a horrible disease. How proper is this thought to deter those persons who have still some reason and shame.

A fourth cause in those addicted to masturbation, is beside these emissions of semen, the frequency of the erections, although imperfect, of which they complain, which exhausts them considerably. Every part which is distended suffers loss of power, and these parts have the most of it to lose; the nervous influence is here more concentrated, but as it becomes dissipated it thus weakens. The other functions are deprived of it and hence they are performed imperfectly; the concurrence of these two causes is attended with dangerous results. Another symptom to which those addicted to masturbation are very much exposed, is a species of paralysis of the genital organs, which is followed by impotence, the want of erections, and simple gonorrhea, because the relaxed parts cause the real semen to escape, as it arrives there and the fluid secreted by the prostate gland dribbles continually, and finally, all the inner membrane of the urethra becomes catarrhal which disposes it to pour out a fluid of the same nature as that of fluor albus in women, a circumstance which is more common than is generally supposed; this affection is not confined to the membrane which lines the nostrils, the throat and lungs, but often attacks all the hollow viscera, and is mistaken because not suspected and badly treated because it is not recognized; we could easily find in reported cases, instances of this disease, treated for another.

An eminent surgeon mentioned to me a man who, addicted by a singular taste for the lowest kind of venereal indulgence, having intercourse only in the corners of the streets, became finally exhausted and affected with severe pains in the kidneys, with emaciation, dryness and paralysis of the legs, which seemed to depend on the position he took in these low connections. He died, after passing six months in bed, in a state to excite pity and horror. Does not this case add a fifth cause of the dangers commonly peculiar to masturbation? When the strength is lost by these two ways at the same time, feebleness ensues in a much greater degree. A person sitting or standing must in order to keep himself in these situations, especially in the first, call a great many muscles into action, and this action weakens the nervous energy. Debilitated persons who cannot stand a moment without feeling feeble, the sick who cannot sit without feeling this also, prove it very evidently. Perhaps in lying down in an extended position, this power is not necessary. It is seen that the same act in one of these attitudes produces more debility than in the other, in the first case, than in the second; and Sanctorius had already indicated the danger of this position: "Usus coitus stando, lædit; nam musculos et eorum utilem perspirationem diminuit."

Other cases which are well attested, furnish a sixth cause which perhaps might appear trivial, but which enlightened physicians consider of some consequence; all living bodies perspire; there is exhaled at every instant by the exhalent vessels of the skin, an extremely thin fluid which amounts to much more than all the other evacuations, at the same time another kind of vessels admit a part of the fluids which surround the body and carry them into the other vessels. These are the *torrens invisibles*, to use the happy expression of Senac, which leave our bodies and enter them again. This absorption has been proved in some cases to be very great. Strong persons perspire most; the weak who have almost no atmosphere, inspire most, and this expired part, or this perspiration of persons in good health contains something nutritious and strengthening, which inspired by another contributes to give strength.

These observations explain how the young woman, with whom David slept, gave him strength; how this same thing has succeeded with other old men to whom it has been advised; and why this weakens the young person who looses it without receiving any thing in exchange, or rather who receives the weak, corrupted and putrid exhalations which are so injurious. A person perspires more during coition than at any other time, because the power of the circulation is quickened. This perspiration is perhaps more active and more volatile than at any other time: it is a real loss, and occurs whenever emissions of semen take place, from whatever cause, since it depends on the agitation attending it. In coition it is reciprocal, and the one inspires, what the other expires. This exchange has been verified by certain observations. In masturbation there is a loss without this reciprocal benefit.

In observing the effect of the passions, we discover a seventh difference between those who have sexual intercourse, and those who practice onanism: a difference which is disadvantageous to the latter. The exhilaration of the mind, which must be distinguished from that purely corporeal pleasure, which man possesses in common with animals, and which is very different, aids digestion, animates the circulation, favors all the functions, re-establishes the strength and sustains it. If they be connected with the pleasures of love, it contributes to restore that energy which otherwise might have been lost: this is proved by observation. Sanctorius has remarked that "After excessive coition with a woman one loves and desires, we do not feel the lassitude which should result from this excess, because the exhilaration experienced in the mind, increases the strength of the heart, favors the functions and repairs what had been lost." It is on this principle that Venette, in a work where we find a well written chapter on the dangers of an excessive indulgence in the pleasures of sexual intercourse, states that connection with a beautiful female exhausts less, than with an ugly one. Beauty has charms which expand the heart and increase the spirits. We must believe with St. Chrysostome that in an unnatural excitement the crime is greater on this side, than on the other. But can it be doubted that nature has attached more delight to pleasure procured in accordance with her designs, than in opposition to them.

Loin des plaisirs que le remords doit suivre.
Miseri quorum gaadia crimen habent.

An eighth, and last cause which increases the dangers of onanism, is the horror of the conscience with which it is followed, when its consequences have opened the eyes of those addicted to it, to the crime and its dangers. If there be any exposed to the horrors of conscience they are those addicted to onanism. When the vail is withdrawn, the picture of their conduct appears in the most hideous light; they have been guilty of a crime which must be punished by Divine justice, and of one which is punished with death by Pagans.

Hoc nihil esse putas : ocetus est, mihi crede, sed ingens
Quantum vix animo consipis ipse tuo.
—Mart.

The shame which follows them infinitely increases their misery. Such is the degree of dissipation in some places, that females of ill fame are considered almost a benefit; the most guilty with these make no mystery of it, and do not think they subject themselves to contempt. But where is the onanist who dares avow his infamy? And is not this concealment of crime a proof of guilt? How many have died for not daring to reveal the cause of their disease? In how many letters in the work, Onania do we find this expression: "I had rather die than see you after this confession." One is in fact, and should be more ready to excuse him who, seduced by that propensity engraved by nature on all hearts, and which is designed to perpetuate the species, is wrong only in not keeping within the bounds prescribed by the law and by health. It is when a man is actuated by passions that he forgets himself, and we are much more ready to forgive him, than one who sins against every law, the opinions of men, and the order of nature. Knowing how much he must be degraded in society should it be known, he is constantly tormented by the idea. "It seems," says one of these criminals to me in the same letter we have quoted above, "as if every one reads in my countenance the infamous cause of my disease, and this thought unfits me for society." They become sad and melancholy, (instances of this have been shown in the fourth section of this work,) and are affected by all the evils produced by their long continuance, without having, which is frightful to a criminal, any pretense of justification or one consoling reflection. What are the effects of melancholy sadness? Relaxation of the fibres, languid circulation, indigestion, emaciation, obstructions occasioned by these alterations which seem to be particularly the effects of sadness, effusions of the fluids which result from these alterations: the bile-ducts close, says Senac, and the bile is carried into every part of the body; spasms, convulsions, paralysis, pains, increase of anguish: all these may ensue.

It is useless to be more diffuse on the peculiar dangers of masturbation. They are too real: we pass to consider the mode of cure.

ARTICLE III.

TREATMENT.

SECTION IX.

TREATMENT PROPOSED BY OTHER PHYSICIANS.

In some diseases we are almost certain that our remedies will be successful. Those which result from exhaustion, from excesses in venery, and still more particularly from masturbation, do not belong to this class; and our prognostic when it has arrived to a certain degree, is unfavorable. Hippocrates has foretold death. "This is a bad disease," says Boerhaave, "I have frequently seen it, and I have never been able to cure it." Van Swieten treated the patient of whom he speaks, three years without success. I have seen them die miserably from this disease. There are other patients whom I have not been even able to relieve. Notwithstanding, these examples should not discourage us: some have been more successful. Some cases successfully treated, are found in the treatise, *Onania*, reported by physicians.

Where Hippocrates gives the description quoted above, he points out the treatment. "When the patient is found in this condition," says he, "use fomentations to the whole body, then give an emetic, and after it, a cathartic to purge the head, and after this another to purge the lower parts. It is particularly necessary to commence this cure in the spring. After the purgatives give a little whey or asses milk; then cow's milk for forty days. During the use of the milk no animal food should be taken, but at night it may be thickened with barley-flour. Having finished the use of the milk, some of the most tender meats may be allowed, commencing with a very small quantity and gradually increasing it. The patient should avoid for one year all debauchery, all acts of venery and other immoderate exercise; his walks should be so directed as to avoid the cold and the sun."

We see that Hippocrates commenced the cure by vomiting and purging. His authority does not however make it a law; for this practice would be injurious in the greatest number of cases. It is easy to get out of this embarrassment by remarking that he prescribed purgatives only with a view to give a proper direction to the fluids which he supposod to be thrown from the head and spinal marrow; and that in another place he mentions patients from excesses in venery, among those to whom he did not give purgatives, "because they not only are unable to do good, but may do harm." This last must be considered a general rule; the first forms an exception, an exception founded on a theory now known to be erroneous, which should therefore be rejected.

In Hoffman's desertation, so often cited, are two cases which should make us very careful in the use of emetics, and which we shall mention. A man, fifty years old, long addicted to sexual intercourse, became languid, thin, and consumptive; his sight was sensibly diminished; he saw every thing dimly; at this period he took an emetic to prevent the fever, which he feared after a long use of bacon; it affected his head and rendered him totally blind. A public prostitute, whose sight was obscured whenever she had connection with a man, having taken an emetic, became blind.

Boerhaave seems inclined to mention the difficulties of cure rather than the remedies. "There is but little chance of cure; milk passes too easily: excercise on horseback does not benefit patients with this disease, and they complain that these remedies weaken them: in fact exercise causes a more abundant discharge of semen, and also weakens them. In the morning the patient is bathed in sweat, and enfeebled by sleep; they cannot bear aromatics, the effects of which are also dangerous. The only remedies in this case are nutritious food, moderate excercise, foot baths, and careful frictions."

Among the consultations of this great man, annexed by Haller, to his addition of them, is one for a man who was impotent.

"In a man thirty years old, the genital organs were so weakened that the semen escaped at the commencement of an erection, for it was never perfect, and the semen was not ejaculated, but escaped by drops, and hence his potency, memory, stomach, kidneys, and legs, were totally enfeebled."

Boerhaave affirms these diseases are very difficult to cure; they are never seen except when so weak that remedies are ineffectual. The following treatment may be tried;

1. A dry and light diet, composed of birds, mutton, veal, beef or kid, roasted rather than boiled; a small quantity of excellent beer, and a little of very nice wine.

2. Much exercise, gradually increased to weariness, and always on an empty stomach.

3. Frictions with warm flannel over the stomach, kidneys, pubis, haunches, and scrotum, made regularly every morning and evening.

4. Every two hours during the day half a drachm of the following.

"R. Terra Japon . . . . dr. iv.
Opopanac . . . . " v.
Cort. Peruv. . . . . " vi.
Cons. Ros. Rub. . . . . oz. i.
Oliban . . . . dr. ii.
Succ. Misce cac. unc. ss. syrup. Kerm. q. s.f. l. a. cond."

"Let him drink immediately half an ounce of the following medicinal wine

"R. Rad carophill mont. . . . . oz. i.
Pæn. Mar. a. a. . . . . oz i.
Cort. rad. cappar. . . . . oz. i. ss.
Tamarisc. a. a. . . . . oz i.
Lign. agalloch. veri. . . . . oz. i.
Vin. gall. alb. . . . . . . lbs. vi. f. l. a. vin. med."

I hoped, added Boerhaave, the patient would be cured after following this prescription two months. But he did not use it and died after a few weeks with malignant dysenteria. What would have been the effect of the remedy? This cannot be told. Zimmermann has written to me that he used it in a case for two months without success.

Hoffman mentions the precautions to be taken, and the remedies to be employed. "We must avoid all remedies not proper for weak persons, and which might weaken them, such as all the astringents, those which are too cold, as preparations of lead, nitre, acids, and particularly narcotics; they are all injurious in cases of this kind, and unfortunately they are frequently used.

The end to be proposed is to re-establish the strength by restoring the natural tone of the fibres. The warm, volatile, aromatic remedies, those which have a strong and pleasant odor are not proper; mild nourishment which tends to restore the gelatinous substance carried off by the evacuations are requisite, as rich broths of chicken, veal, beef, with a little wine, lemon juice, and salt. Those remedies which favor the perspiration, and which restore the languid state of the fibres, may be used with success."

In another consultation for a person addicted to masturbation, he ordered a pint of asses milk diluted with one third of Seltzer water, to be taken every morning.

It would be useless to enumerate here the advice or remarks of other authors. We shall merely mention a very useful case given in a desertation of Westprime, who relates fourteen cases all of which are interesting.

W. Conybeare, thirty years old, for six years had his sight so much obscured, without any apparent affection of the eye, that he saw objects dimly. He had been successively in three of the best London hospitals, St. Thomas', St. Bartholomew's, and St. George's; and finally he remained two years in ours. Every where else after other remedies were used, salivation was employed to cure this kind of gutta serena. The physicians were wearied and the patient discouraged. Interrogating him strictly on his disease, he told me, that he occasionally felt a pain along the dorsal spine, especially, when he stooped to take up any thing; that his legs were so weak that he could scarcely stand for a moment without support, and that he was affected with vertigo; his memory was so much enfeebled that he sometimes appeared stupid; I saw he was extremely emaciated. All this made me suspect that gutta serena was only a symptom of a frightful disease, and, that the patient was affected with *tabes dorsalis.* I anxiously inquired if he ever indulged in onanism which destroys the nervous system. After much delay he blushingly admitted it. I ordered him to take two murcurial pills, three grains each at night, and the morning after an ounce of Sulph. Magnesia, and to repeat four times in fifteen days. At the end of that time I put him on a milk diet. At the same time he was rubbed three times a week. After this he returned to the country in much better health than when he left. I then advised him the use of the cold bath: he took one every two days for three weeks at 8 o'clock, A. M. fasting. This course re-established his health to such an extent that he wished to resume his occupation which was that of a baker, but I advised him to change it lest inhaling the flour might produce dangerous effects, as his nerves were yet weak.

Stehelin relieved the patient mentioned above by baths, mineral tonics, and aperient broths.

The principal remedies in Onania, are secrets. We see generally that no laxative is employed and that tonics are their base. Their action produces no sensible effects, yet they are said to strengthen the genital parts, impart to them new power, favor the secretion of semen, and powerfully recruit exhausted nature; in a word they perform whatever is desired, like all other quack medicines. A third remedy termed the restoring portion is also said to be very efficacious; in fact, if we are to believe all the testimonies in favor of these medicines they are very valuable. Besides these he also prescribes some formulas; one is a portion composed of amber, aromatics, and some other remedies of the same class; a second is a liniment composed of essential oils and acrid tinctures: both of these compositions seem to us too stimulating; and as we have had no experience with them they will be omitted. He mentions two others which seem more proper.

R. Flor. siccat. lamii . . . . mpl. vi.
Rad. cyper. et Galang. aa . . . . oz. ii.
Rad. Bistort . . . . " i.
Rad. osmund. regal . . . . " ii.
Flor. ros. rubr. mpl. . . . . " iii.

Sicissa tuf. mixt. cum aquæ quar. VIII. ad quartæ part. evaporat. coquant. Every day a quart to be taken.

R. Plumbi Acet.
Zinci Sulph.
Alum. aa.

> Agr. Chalyb. Fabror. pt. iss. per dies decem igne arenæ digerantur: add. spir. vin. camph. cochl. III. For an injection.

In a work called *Precis de Medicine pratique* by Lieutaud, physician at Paris, are some very good views on this disease; his name is already distinguished among anatomists and physiologists, and this work entitles him to a high rank among practitioners. The chapters relating to dorsal consumption, are entitled *Calor morbosus*, which disease is very frequent and is mentioned by no one; it is often treated very badly as we have mentioned, and its symptoms, nature and treatment were first developed by Lieutaud; *vires exhaustæ* and *anæmia*, which may be translated, a loss of blood; they form a very interesting chapter written entirely by the author.

Lewis, whose work we could not procure before our first edition was printed, enlarges most on the treatment. I am pleased to see that we perfectly agree in our views and employ the same remedies, especially the cinchona and cold baths, which agreement seems to favor the mode followed by both of us. I shall mention here only two aphorisms which include the substance of his treatment. I shall use some of his explanations in the next section to confirm my own practice.

"The cure of this disease depends," says he, "on two things, what must be done and what must be avoided; and remedies have no power unless we attend to the non-naturals, to all parts of the regimen. A healthy pure air is of the utmost importance. The diet should be nutritious but not stimulating. The sleep should not be too long and at proper hours. The patient should exercise moderately, especially on horseback. If the natural evacuations be irregular, they must be regulated. The patient should endeavor to amuse himself by company or innocent pleasures. All the remedies should be drawn from two classes, the tonic and balsamic."

He recommends instead of tea, which he says is very injurious to the nervous system, an infusion of balm or of mint, adding to each cup a table-spoonful of a balsamic mixture composed of cream and the yolk of eggs, beaten with two or three drops of the oil of canella, which makes a very pleasant drink; this remedy is truly balsamic and tonic. We will here remark that preparations of lead are among the tonics advised by Lewis; it is our duty to mention that notwithstanding his authority, and that of some other respectable physicians, the internal use of these preparations are poisonous; we have seen the worst effects from them, and the impudence of quacks furnishes too many cases. If like some other poisons it must be retained, its administration should be confided to those who know its virtues and its dangers, and should not be recommended in popular works without caution.

We shall conclude this section by giving the treatment of Stork. It is very simple and efficacious. In comparing all these methods, we see they are all founded on the same principles, that they all tend to the same end, and that they all employ very similar means. This coincidence is in favor of our treatment and inspires us with confidence. "We begin," says Stork "with succulent broths. Rice and barley in milk or broth, and milk are very useful; but little must be taken at a time, and frequently repeated. If, as sometimes happens when the disease has made great progress, this food produces pain, the patient must be nursed, which has sometimes proved very beneficial. Power and action are restored to the relaxed fibres by the use of wine, with iron, cinchona, and canella; when the patient is strong enough to walk, the country air is extremely useful.

SECTION X.

TREATMENT BY THE AUTHOR.

It is difficult to determine the cause of some diseases, and therefore, to point out the indications and regulate their treatment, which however are sometimes easily cured when these are obtained. This is not the case however with tabes dorsalis. The disease and the cause are known, "it is," says Lewis, "a peculiar species of consumption, the proximate cause of which is general debility of the nervous system." The indications are evident, and there can be no discrepancy in regard to the essential part of the treatment; but the best mode is frequently neglected, and therefore we shall be very minute in the details. The general relaxation of the fibres, the weakness of the nervous system, and the alteration in the fluids, are the causes of the disease. It involves all parts, and we must restore to them their tone; this is the only indication. Its particulars depend on the different parts enfeebled: but as the same remedies are useful for all, we shall omit them here. Those who are perfectly ignorant of medicine, but who talk more than the scientific, think this is easily accomplished by tonics and nutritious food, so abundant in our shops; but sad experience has taught the most distinguished physicians that it is very difficult.

It is very easy, says Gotter, to reduce the strength, but difficult to restore it. This will be easily understood, when we reflect that the food and the remedies are only instruments used by nature to restore all losses in the system, and remove all derangements which supervene. What is nature? It is the aggregate of the vital powers distributed throughout the body, in such a manner as to produce harmonious and regular action. When these powers are nearly exhausted, nature then is in fault; her energies are feeble, and give her as many materials as you please, she is not in a condition to use them. The food does not invigorate, the medicines do not act. I have seen the stomach so enfeebled, that it had no more powers of digestion than a wooden vessel: sometimes the different articles taken are arranged in it according to the laws of their specific gravities: and finally when a new dose irritates the stomach by its weight, it is rejected by a slight effort; sometimes by continuing there a long time, they are changed and vomited in the state they would be in had they been left to decay in a silver or porcelain vessel. What must be expected from food, in a case of this kind?

All are not so much exhausted. In some the powers are weakened and not entirely destroyed: there is then some assistance to be derived from food and medicine.

The feebleness produced by masturbation renders the choice of tonics difficult, since those which irritate and excite the venereal propensities should be strictly avoided. It is a law of the animal mechanism, the laws of which are so different from those of inanimate nature, that when the vital actions are increased, the increase is greatest in the parts most susceptible of them; in those addicted to Onanism the effect of irritating remedies will be most evident in the genital organs, and the dangerous consequences of this effect cannot make us too careful in regard to the means employed. What then must they be? We shall mention this after the regimen. I shall follow in this detail, the common division into six *non-naturals*, the air, food, sleep, exercise, natural evacuations, and passions.

AIR

The air has the same, and even more influence upon us, than water has upon fishes. Those who know how far this influence extends, will perceive how necessary it is for patients to breathe one air in preference to another. Those who have ever entered a close chamber, breathed the air from marshes in hot weather, lived in low and confined places, passed from a populous city into the country, breathed the air at the rising of the sun, or at noon, before or after a shower, all these will understand the influence the air has on the health:

"Temperie coeli corpusque animusque juvatur." —Ovid.

The weak have more need of pure air than others. It is a remedy which acts without the concurrence of nature, without employing its energies; it is therefore a remedy which should not be neglected. A dry and temperate air is generally most proper; a moist or hot air should be avoided. I know a patient who is completely exhausted by excessive heat, and whose health in summer varies according to the heat of the weather. Cold is not so pernicious, which is a necessary consequence, since heat relaxes the fibres which are already too much so. When the Carribeans are affected with paralysis, in consequence of those spasmodic colics[39] to which they are subject, arid they cannot be sent to the warm baths in the north of Jamaica, they go to a colder climate, and this change is always very favorable. Another essential quality of the air is, that it has not lost, by circulating in inhabited places, all its vivifying power; hence it may be called the vital spirit which is as necessary to plants as to animals. Such is the air in an open country where vegetation flourishes.

If the patient, says Aræteus, lives near fountains and rivulets, the exhalations from them, and the delight inspired by these objects, reanimates the soul, and imparts new strength. The air of the city, constantly inspired and expired, is loaded with infectious vapors, and not only possesses less exhilarating effects but is filled with injurious particles; that of the country contains the two opposite properties; it is pure and is loaded with the most volatile, the most pleasant, the most cordial parts of the plants, and with that of the earth which is also salubrious. But it would be useless to reside in a healthy air, if you do not breathe it in bed-chambers, which if not constantly renewed, is nearly the same in all; there is but little change in passing from a close chamber in the city, to one in the country. The salubrity of a healthy atmosphere, is not enjoyed except in the open air. If infirmities or weakness prevent one from going out, the chamber should be aired several times a day, not merely by opening a door or a window, but by causing a circulation of air through the room. Every disease requires this precaution, but then it is proper to guard the patient against a too great impression from it, which is always very easy.

It is also extremely important to breathe the morning air; those who deprive themselves of it by remaining in a close atmosphere, voluntarily renounce the best, and perhaps the most strengthening of all remedies. The freshness of night, restores the vivifying power, and the dew which gradually evaporates after being loaded with the perfumes of the flowers on which it had rested, is truly medicinal. We float on the breath of the blooming plants, and constantly inhale their delicious fragrance. A feeling of health and of freshness, of strength and appetite, is one proof of the invigorating powers of nature, which may be tested by any one. We have very recently seen the most marked effects on some invalids, especially on those who are hypocondriacal; they are very conscious that on breathing the morning air, they are much more gay the rest of the day, and their attendants cannot be mistaken in regard to the time they arise from bed. The importance of this fact, in respect to those affected with dorsal consumption, who are so often hypocondriacal, is easily recognized. The return of their gayety alone demonstrates an improvement in their health.

FOOD

The choice of food should be regulated by these two rules, first, to take no food except that which contains much nutrition in a small compass, and which is easy of digestion. This is an aphorism of Sanctorius: *Coitus immoderatus postulet cibos paucas et boni nutrimenli.* Second, to avoid all those things which are acrid. It is important that the stomach should not be oppressed with an improper diet, for if the stomach be dilated with too much food, it is daily weakened. Farther, if it be too much filled, persons in feeble health are affected with pain, feebleness, and melancholy, which aggravate their symptoms. These two inconveniences will be prevented by choosing such food as we have mentioned, and by taking a little at a time and repeating it often. It is necessary that the food should be easily digested; the stomach not being in a state to act upon crude substances, its powers which are extremely languid, would be entirely destroyed by food which is too hard or difficult to digest.

Upon these principles we could form a catalogue of articles, which are proper in these cases and of those which should be avoided. In the last class are all meats naturally hard and indigestible, as pork, and flesh of old animals, salted and smoked meats, which are too acrid. All those which are too fat, and any other fatty substances, relax the fibres of the stomach, and diminish the action of the digestive juices, which are already too weak; they remain undigested, dispose to obstructions, and by continuing in the stomach become so acrid, that they cause pain, restlessness, want of sleep, and fever. In fact, there is nothing against which persons affected with dyspepsia, should guard more carefully than fatty substances; unleavened pastry, especially when mixed with fat, is another kind of food beyond the powers of a deranged stomach. Potherbs produce distention, and at the same time obstruct the circulation in the adjacent parts; they are likewise injurious; such are generally all kinds of cabbage, beans, and vegetables, especially those which have an acrid odor and taste, which last quality renders them injurious, besides causing flatulence.

Fruits which are salutary in acute and inflammatory diseases, in obstructions, especially in those of the liver, and in several other maladies, are improper in these cases; they debilitate, relax, and enervate the powers of the stomach: they tend to render the blood more liquid which is already too watery. When badly digested, they ferment in the stomach and intestines, and this fermentation generates an immense quantity of air, which produces enormous distention, and thus absolutely deranges the course of circulation. I have seen this effect very great in a female, in whom, on eating too freely of ripe fruit 24 hours after a very fortunate confinement, the abdomen became tense and livid: she swooned and her pulse became almost imperceptible. Fruits also leave in the primæ viæ an acrid principle, which may cause severe symptoms: and hence they must be avoided. Crude potherbs, vinegar, and verjuice, are attended with the same inconvenience and deserve to be excluded.

Although the catalogue of prohibited articles of food may be long, that of those substances allowed is still longer. It includes all food of young animals, nourished in good situations, and well fed, especially, veal, lamb, beef, chickens, pigeons; guinea-hens, partridges, ducks, and other game, although not absolutely forbidden, are however somewhat inconvenient, and hence ought not to be used daily; the same is true of fish.

Not only should the meats be chosen carefully, but be properly prepared. The best way of cooking, is to roast them at a moderate fire, which preserves their juices and does not dry them, or to stew them in their own gravy. Those which are boiled with a great deal of water, impart all their nutrition to the water; hence they are frequently only fleshy fibres, destitute of nourishment, and filled with water, and are mostly insipid and indigestible.

The more tender the meats, the less should they be cooked in this manner, for which the hard meats alone should be employed in order to draw from them their nourishment.

However carefully the food may be prepared, some persons cannot digest it; hence they must be allowed only the juices, which should be pressed after they are moderately cooked: but as they are easily spoiled, a little of bread, and of lemon juice, or wine must be added; this mixture is the most nutritious which can be used. Some shell-fish stewed in their liquor, may stimulate the taste, and render it still stronger—but they have two inconveniences, they are slightly stimulant, and cause the broth to spoil more quickly, which must be gaurded against. Bread and vegetables, have not the advantage of containing much nutrition in a small space: but they, especially bread, are indispensably necessary to prevent not only the distaste which the use of animal food entirely would produce, but also the putridity which would ensue, if vegetables were not used. Without this precaution, free alkali would soon be developed in the primæ viæ, and be followed by all the disorders which it might produce. I have seen the most severe symptoms occasioned by this regimen in weak persons to whom it was prescribed.

One of the most common symptoms is thirst; the patients are obliged to drink, and drink weakens them: further it does not combine with the fluids, because this mixture depends on the action of the vessels which is very languid: and if from a very common affection in those who take but little excercise, the action of the kidneys is diminished, fluids pass into the cellular tissue, and first form œdemas, and then all kinds of dropsies. These bad consequences may always be prevented by combining an animal with a vegetable diet. The best vegetables are tender roots and herbs, as asparagus. Others although very tender, incommode, because they are too cold: they weaken the powers of the stomach.

The farinaceous[40] substances prepared and cooked in milk, or with broth, form a very nutritious substance: it unites the most nourishing of the animal and vegetable kingdoms, and the mixture prevents the danger of each article of food taken separately. It is easily seen on reading cases with some degree of attention, that diseases are more malignant in the north of Europe than in the central portion. Does not this come from their eating more meat and less vegetables than in the former place?

Our remarks above do not prohibit the occasional use of fruits, which must be of the best kind, and perfectly ripe, and should be used in small quantities; the most watery are most to be avoided.

Eggs are an article of food from the animal kingdom, and are extremely useful; they are very strengthening, and are easily digested, when not cooked too much or too little; for, when the white of the egg is hard, it does not dissolve; it becomes heavy and indigestible and does not nourish: it becomes then an article of food for stomachs which can digest any thing, and not for those of dyspeptic persons. The best mode of eating them is from the shell, or after they have been dipped three or four times in boiling water, or into hot, but not boiling broth. Finally a last article of food, is milk; it contains all desirable qualities, and is free from all objections. It is very simple and is easily digested, and it restores the strength most promptly: being prepared by nature, it cannot be made offensive by any artificial preparation. It is as nutritious as the juice of beef, and does not become putrid; it prevents thirst, being both food and drink: it keeps up all the secretions, and disposes to tranquil sleep. In a word it fulfills all the indications presented by these cases, and Lewis has seen it produce the best effects. Why then is it not employed always? And why is it not substituted for other nourishment? For a special reason, viz. that it sometimes produces an unexpected effect. This is the kind of decomposition to which it is subject. If it be not digested soon, if it remains too long in the stomach, or if the stomach contains substances which hasten its decomposition, it undergoes the same changes, as when out of the body. The butyraceous, the caseous, and the serous portions separate; the whey sometimes causes diarrhea; sometimes it passes off through the urinary passages, or by transpiration, without nourishing the body: if either parts remain in the stomach, they soon molest it, occasion diseases, swellings, nausea, and colics; if one is not incommoded immediately, it is because they pass into the intestines, where they may remain a certain time, without producing any manifest effect: but they there become singularly acrid, and after a certain time, they give rise to symptoms which are dangerous, although they did not appear immediately: hence it may be mentioned as a law, when milk is ordered in severe cases, that if it be the article of food most easily digested, it is also that which if undigested, produces the most severe symptoms. The difficulties found by Boerhaave in its use, have been mentioned above, but however great these may be, the advantages to be derived from it are so important, that all possible means should be used to prevent them. These may be arranged in two classes, attention to regimen, and remedies.

Attention to regimen are, 1st., the choice of milk; whatever the kind selected, the female should be healthy and well fed; 2dly., all crude and cooked fruits, and all acids must be avoided; 3dly., other kinds of food must be taken at long intervals from it; mixtures must not take place; 4thly., but little must be taken at once; 5thly., the stomach, abdomen, and legs, must be kept warm, and 6thly., (which is the most important, as without this all others are useless,) the quantity of other food, even when selected with the greatest care, must be extremely moderate. The stomach should be allowed to rest while the milk is taken; the smallest excess, the least indigestion, leaves in it a principle which immediately corrupts the milk, and sometimes changes the most healthy food into an acrid poison, or at least renders it very injurious.

What milk deserves the preference? To answer this question, we shall not examine the different kinds of milk: it would extend our work too much; at present, only that of the woman, the ass, the goat, and the cow, are employed. Each has its different qualities, and the choice of one of them must be determined by the comparison of those qualities, and the indications presented by the disease. There are but few cases where that of the cow is not preferable to all others. That of the woman is generally considered the most strengthening by the most celebrated physicians, but this opinion rests on a wrong foundation, viz. the use of meat; they not considering at the same time, that of a robust peasant girl is preferred who eats but very little of it, and lives on bread and vegetables. We believe however that it may be used with success; the fine cures performed by it, leave no doubt in regard to its efficacy. But it has one peculiar inconvenience, it must be drawn from the nipple. Galen knew the necessity of this, since he advises those who cannot submit to it, to go like asses to asses' milk. But would not this excite those desires which ought to be forgotten? And would not this expose one to see renewed the adventure of the prince, whose history has been related by Capivaccio? He was supplied with two nurses, and their milk produced so good an effect, that he left them in a condition to furnish fresh milk after a few months, if this was needed.

It is thought that asses' milk is most similar to that of the female, but allow me to say, this is rather an opinion than a fact. It is more serous, and hence it is more relaxing; it is a fatal error to think it is the most strengthening. Daily observation proves the contrary, and not only that it is not the most efficacious, but perhaps the least so. I have not always seen good effects from it nor am I the only one. It seems, says Haller, to me, that asses' milk rarely does what is required of it; a want of utility is a great defect in a remedy, on which the care of severe diseases depends. Hoffman advised it in those cases where there were both exhaustion and desire.

Before leaving the subject of food, we might mention the advice of Horace: it is not to make mixtures.

> ————Nam variæ res
> Ut noceant homini, credas, memor illius escæ;
> Quæ simplex olim tibi sederit; at simul assis
> Miscueris elixa, simul conchylia turdis,
> Dulcia se in bilem vertent, stomachoque tumultum
> Lenta feret pituita.

We need not insist upon the impossibility of very different articles of food being perfectly digested. The mixture is one of the causes which ruin the constitution of the most vigorous, and destroy the feeble; it cannot be avoided too carefully.

Another attention also necessary, and neglected in almost an equal degree, is perfect mastication: this is required by the strongest stomachs, and cannot be dispensed with without sensibly affecting them. Much observation is necessary to imagine the importance of perfect mastication to the health. I have seen the most stubborn diseases and debility of the stomach removed by attention to this particular alone. I have seen on the other side, persons in health, become diseased when their teeth failed, and mastication was imperfect: and they were restored to health only when their teeth were entirely lost, and their gums became hard enough to fulfill their functions.

These details, these precautions, and privations, are expressed in one verse of Procopius:

> Vivre selon nos lois, c'est vivre miserable.

But can one pay too dearly for health? How well paid are we for sacrifices by the pleasure of enjoying it, and by the delights which it imparts to every moment of life. "Without health," says Hippocrates, "there is no pleasure; honors, riches, and all worldly goods are useless." Farther, these sacrifices are much less than they are thought. For, we can adduce several who at first, had no difficulty in renouncing the variety of dishes, in order to confine themselves to simple regimen. This is indicated by nature, and is best adapted to organs in health. A healthy palate which has its natural sensibility, can taste only of the simple meats, and the complex cannot be endured; it finds in the least savory food, a taste which is imperceptible in blunted organs. Thus those who return to a simple diet on account of their health, although with some disgust, may rest assured, that they will find in this food, pleasures which they did not expect. A correct ear distinguishes a slight difference between two tones, which escapes a less sensible ear. The same is true with the nerves of the organ of taste; when delicate, they perceive the slightest variety in tastes, and are sensible to them. Among those who drink water, are some to whom it is as pleasant as the choicest wine. Finally, when we do not expect to follow a particular regimen with pleasure, (as it is easy to pursue that mentioned by me,) the satisfaction of knowing that we fulfill a duty, is a very pressing motive with those who know the value of an approving conscience.

The drinks are a part of the regimen almost as important as the food.

We must omit all those which may increase the debility and relaxation, diminish the slight digestive powers which remain, render the humors acrid, and cause a greater irritability in the nervous system. All warm drinks have the first effect; they all coexist in tea; coffee possesses the last two, and should therefore be strictly avoided. Thiery, the author of a work above all praise, and of which those interested in the progress of medicine are impatient for the continuation, has pointed out the danger of these fluids, in a sketch which would probably disgust those who take them with most pleasure.

Spirituous liquors which seem at first view to be proper, inasmuch as they produce precisely the opposite effect of warm water, the danger of which they diminish if added in small quantities, have other great inconveniences for which they should be rejected, or at least should be used very rarely. Their action is too violent, and too transient, and if they sometimes strengthen, the debility which follows is greater than before their use; they also harden the papillæ of the stomach, which lose the degree of sensibility necessary to an appetite and remove from the digestive fluids, that degree of fluidity necessary to aid this sensation; thus those who drink spirit, are insensible to it. "Those persons," says the illustrious author whom we have cited, "who drink liquors every day after dinner, in order to remedy the difficulties of digestion, can do no better than take them, if they wish to destroy the digestive powers."

The best drink is very pure water, mixed with an equal quantity of wine, which is neither smoky nor acid; the first irritates the nervous system, and slightly rarifies the fluids: this distends the vessels and makes them more loose, and renders the fluids more valuable; the second weakens the powers of digestion, irritates and increases the quantity of the urine, which exhausts the patients. The best wines are those which contain alcohol, and salts, and more of earths and oil. Such are some red wines, of Burgundy, the Rhone, Neuf-Chatel, the old white wines of Grave, those of Pontac, the Spanish, and Portuguese; those of the Canaries, and when they can be procured, the Tokay wines are more salubrious, and more pleasant than any other. For common use there are none preferable to the wine of Neuf-Chatel.

In those places where water is not good, it may be corrected by filtration, or by infusing in it some pleasant aromatics, as cannella, annis, and lemon peel.

Common beer is injurious. Rum, which is properly an extract of grain, both nutritious and strengthening, may perhaps be very useful: it possesses some alcohol, invigorates as much as wine, and nourishes more: it may be used for meat and drink.

Among the useful drinks we must mention chocolate, which perhaps more properly belongs to the class of food: cocoa contains more nutrition, and being mixed with sugar and aromatics, it is not so injurious as an oily substance. "Chocolate with milk," says Lewis, "taken in a small quantity, so as not to overload the stomach, is an excellent breakfast for consumptive persons." I know a child three years old, who was in the last stage of this disorder, and was given up by his physician; his mother gave him chocolate in small quantities and frequently, and he was thus cured; it is true that this food cannot be too much recommended to invalids. It would be very injurious to several.

As a general remark, great quantities of any drink should be avoided: It enfeebles the digestive powers, by relaxing the stomach, it injures the digestive juices, and precipitates the food before it is digested; it relaxes all the parts, it dissolves all the humors, and disposes to the formation of urine and debilitating sweats. I have seen diseases produced by atony diminish considerably, without any other remedy than the omission of part of the drink.

SLEEP

Our remarks on sleep may be reduced to three heads: its duration, the time of sleeping, and the necessary precautions for enjoying tranquil slumber.

Seven or eight hours of sleep are enough for an adult; there is danger in sleeping more and remaining longer in bed: this produces the same disorders as too much sleep. If any class of persons may sleep a longer time, it is those who exercise very much through the day, but they do not indulge in it, on the contrary, it is those who lead a sedentary life; thus they should never exceed this length of time, unless they are so feeble that they cannot sit up for a long time. In this case, they must lie down as much as possible. "The less one sleeps," says Lewis " the more mild and refreshing is the slumber."

The night air is more injurious than that of the day, and invalids are more susceptible of its influence at night than in the morning; while confined to a small quantity of air, which must be corrupt, we must devote to sleep that period of time, when the air is least healthy, and when the respiration of this unhealthy air would be most injurious to us. Thus we must retire early and rise early in the morning: this precept is so well known, that perhaps it may seem trivial to repeat it, but it is so much neglected, and its importance seems to be so much overlooked, that it is very excusable to suppose it unknown, and to insist upon its importance, particularly to valetudinarians[41]. "If we retire at 10 o'clock, and one ought never to sit up longer," these are Lewis's expressions, "we ought to rise between four and five o'clock, and in winter at six or seven. It is absolutely necessary to forbid those affected with this disorder, to pass the morning in bed." He even thinks it proper that one should be accustomed to rise after the first sleep, and asserts that however painful this custom may be at first, it soon becomes easy and pleasant.. Several instances prove this advice to be good: there are several valetudinarians who feel well on awaking from their first sleep, but are very much indisposed if they sleep again; they are sure of passing a good day, if they arise after their first sleep.

The sleep is disturbed whenever there is a cause of irritation, we should therefore endeavor to prevent them.

The three most important circumstances to be attended to are,—1st., not to be in a warm atmosphere, and not to be too much or too slightly covered. 2d., not to lie down with cold feet, which is a very common thing with invalids, and is injurious for several reasons. In this respect the rule of Hippocrates should be observed exactly, to sleep in a cool place, and be carefully covered. 3d., and which is still more important, not to retire with a full stomach; nothing disturbs the sleep so much as indigestion during the night. Debility, weariness, and incapacity of body and mind, the next day, are the inevitable consequences."

——————Vides ut pallidus omnis
Cœna desurgat dubia? quin corpus onustum
Hesternis vitiis animum quoque degravat una,
Atque affigit humo divinæ particularn auræ. —Hor.

Nothing on the contrary contributes more to a calm and constant sleep, than a light supper. Freshness, agility, and gayety, the next day are the consequences.

> Alter, ubi dicto citius curata sopori
> Membra dedit, vegetus proscripta ad munia surgit.
> —Hor.

Lewis says, and very rationally, that the period of sleep, is one of nutrition and not of digestion, thus he requires of his patients the greatest strictness in regard to suppers; he prohibits, and very properly, meat at evening, he only permits a little milk, and some slices of bread, and that two hours before retiring, in order that the first digestion may be finished before going to sleep. The Atcantes who are famous for never tasting animal food, and never eat any thing which ever had life, were famous for the tranquillity of their sleep, and were ignorant of dreams.

EXERCISE

Exercise is absolutely necessary, it is a task for debilitated persons to take it, and if they are melancholy it is very difficult to induce them to exert themselves. Nothing however tends more to increase all the bad consequences attendant upon debility, than want of exercise; the fibres of the stomach vessels and intestines, are loose, the fluids are stagnated in every part, because the solids have not the power to impart to them the necessary motion, hence effusions, obstructions, and congestions ensue, nutrition and secretions are arrested, the blood remains watery, the strength diminishes, and all the symptoms of the disease increase. Exercise prevents all these evils, by increasing the powers of the circulation, all the functions take place as if there was real strength, which is soon given by a regularity in the functions; thus the effects of exercise are to increase the strength. Another advantage independent of increasing the circulation, is the change of scene; a person who takes no exercise is soon wearied of the scene around him; a person in exercising constantly changes it; exercise may take the place of remedies, but no remedy can supply the want of exercise.

The fatigue in the first days exhausts the courage of many patients, but if they have strength to overcome the first obstacle, they would perceive that it was only the first step which was trying. I have been astonished to see, to what extent those who have not been accustomed to it, acquired strength by exercise. I have seen persons who were fatigued in walking round a garden, gain so much in a few weeks, as to be able to walk six miles, and feel well on their return.

Walking is not the only kind of exercise favorable, that on horseback is much better for those who are very weak, or for those in whom the viscera of the abdomen and chest are affected; where there is still more debility, riding in a coach is still better, provided it is not too easy: when the weather does not allow one to go out, the patient should exercise in the house, or engage in some slightly laborious occupation, or in some exercise which affects the whole body equally.

The return of appetite, of sleep, and of gayety, are the

necessary consequence of this remedy; but we must be careful not to take violent exercise soon after eating, and not to eat when warm; exercise should be taken before evening, and we should rest some moments afterward.

EVACUATIONS

The evacuations are deranged as well as the other functions, and their derangement increases the disorder of the machine: they must be attended to and remedied early. The evacuations which principally demand our attention, are the dejections, the urine, the transpirations, and the mucus. The best mode of preventing them, or restoring them to their natural state, is to attend to our rules of regimen; when these are correctly followed the dejections (the greater or less degree in regularity, of which is the barometer of the better or worse state of digestion), are regular.

That most important to be favored is transpiration, which is daily deranged in feeble persons. It is easily assisted by rubbing the skin with a flesh brush or flannel: when it is very languid, the best way of preserving it is to cover the whole body with flannel; one should avoid being too much dressed, for fear of sweating, which always injures transpiration. The part to be most protected by every one, and by invalids particularly, are the feet. This precaution which is so easy, would not be neglected if its importance to the whole system were known. Frequent cold of the feet causes the most serious chronic diseases; there are a great many persons in whom it soon produces very bad effects; but those particularly who are subject to diseases of the chest, to colics, or obstructions, cannot guard too much against these dangers. The priests, who always walked with bare feet on the pavements of the temples, were often attacked with violent colics.

The saliva is sometimes very abundant in feeble persons; the relaxation of the salivary organs, disposes them to this copious secretion. If the sick persons spit continually, two evil consequences ensue; 1st, they are weakened by this evacuation. 2d, this fluid so necessary to the digestion, which is imperfect without it, is deficient, and hence it is painful. We have already mentioned the dangers of dyspepsia, and hence we need not speak more fully on those of an evacuation which renders it so. For this reason Lewis absolutely prohibits smoking to his patients, as this, among other inconveniences disposes to an abundant flow of saliva, by irritating the salivary glands.

May not the inspiration made by one person from another of which we have spoken before, be mentioned here as a means of cure? Capio Vacchio thought it useful for his patient to sleep between his two nurses, and very probably the inspiration from their expiration, contributed as much as the milk to re-establish his strength. Eeridoes, the cotemporary of Capio Vacchio, and instructor of Forestius, who has mentioned this case, advised a young man who was affected with marasmus, to drink asses' milk, and to sleep with his nurse who was extremely healthy, and in the flower of her age; this advice was attended with good effects, and was discontinued only when the sick patient avowed, that he could no longer resist his inclinations. A useful remedy might be preserved, and the danger of it prevented by keeping the sexes distinct.

PASSIONS

We have already mentioned an intimate connection of the mind with the body; we have stated how much influence the healthy condition of the first had upon the second; the sad effects of melancholy have been stated; hence it is almost useless to add that disagreeable affections of the mind cannot be too much avoided, and it is of the utmost importance to keep it composed in all diseases, and particularly in those which like tabes dorsalis, dispose of themselves to melancholy. But the patients are frequently pleased with this symptom of their illness, and we cannot induce them to make efforts to conquer it: further we must not be deceived and imagine we have only to order them to be gay to make them so; laughter cannot come when commanded, any more than it can be restrained, and it is as impossible to avoid being sad, as it is to have an attack of fever or of the tooth-ache. All that we can ask of the patient is, that he should employ remedies against sadness, as he uses them against other symptoms: these remedies are not so much an intercourse with society, which we have seen is disagreeable on certain accounts, as a change of scene. The constant succession of objects, form a succession of ideas, which distract the mind, and hence this is what is required.

Nothing is more pernicious to persons who think upon one thing, than idleness and inactivity. Nothing is more pernicious to patients in this disorder, than laziness and being alone. Exercise and working in the country are highly advantageous. Lewis wishes them to avoid if possible, all but their own sex. The patient should never be absolutely alone, and should never be allowed to reflect; no reading or any employment of mind should be permitted, these, he says, are causes which exhaust the spirits, and retard the cure. I do not agree with him; reading should be permitted, but they should not be allowed to read for a long time, on account of the feebleness of their sight, but every thing which demands mental application should be forbidden: and all those should be interdicted which bring to mind those ideas which ought to be forgotten: but there are books which without demanding the attention very much, and without bringing to mind dangerous images, agreeably distract them, and prevent the terrible dangers of ennui.

REMEDIES

I shall follow the same order as in the preceding article, and shall mention the remedies to be avoided, before those to be used. I have already stated the first class of those to be excluded, the warm and volatile remedies which irritate. A second class are the opposite, and also very injurious are evacuants. We have already mentioned that the patient was exhausted by sweating, salivation, and abundant discharge of urine. We shall not mention these evacuations again. We know that all remedies which excite them must be avoided. We have now to examine bleeding and evacuations of the primæ viæ. The indication being to restore the strength, to judge of proper remedies, we have only to inquire of these evacuations and fulfill the indication. I shall be brief; there are two cases where bleeding re-establishes the strength, either when the blood has become dense from inflammation, which renders it improper for its uses, and promptly destroys the strength. This is the disease of vigorous and muscular men in whom the circulation is strong: precisely the contrary is true of our patients, and bleeding can only injure them. "Every drop of blood," says Gilchrist, "is precious to consumptive persons; the assimilating power which renews it is destroyed, and they have only what is necessary to maintain the very feeble circulation." Lobb, who knew the effect of evacuants is positive: "in bodies," says he, "who have only the necessary quantity of blood, if this is diminished by bleeding or by other evacuations the strength is diminished, the secretions are disturbed, and several diseases are produced." The manner in which Senac speaks of bleeding excludes it still more positively in this case. "If the dense or red matter is deficient, bleedings are useless or pernicious, they ought not then to be employed in weak persons where there is but little blood, and it is then when only a fluid which scarcely tinges linen or water comes from the vessels." We have already seen that this is the state of blood in those addicted to onanism; and it is generally so in feeble persons. Let those who undertake to cure by bleeding, compare their method with the precepts founded on the most enlightened theory; the most numerous and best practical observations, the foundations upon which I form it, and let them judge the success which they must expect.

Purgatives strengthen either when there is so much forced matter within the alimentary canal, that the functions of all the viscera are impeded, or when putrid substances exist in the stomach or primæ viæ, which generally cause great debility. In these cases we may employ purgatives, if they are not contra indicated, if there be no other mode of emptying the alimentary canal, or when there is no danger of evacuating them suddenly. These three conditions rarely exist in consumptive persons, in whom the weakness and debility of the primæ viæ always contra indicate emetics and purgatives generally. Another mode to procure evacuations, is to employ those tonics which are not astringent; there are a great number of bitters, which by restoring the tone to the organs, produce the double good effect of digesting what can be digested, and of rejecting the remainder. Finally there is rarely danger in not evacuating the bowels promptly; this danger sometimes exists in acute diseases: the acridity of the materials which is augmented by the heat, and the great reaction of the fibres may cause violent symptoms, which never occur in diseases of debility, in which purgatives are by no means as necessary, and are, as we have said, very frequently contra indicated. Debility and want of action aid the causes of the accumulation of fæces; when these are discharged by a purgative the effect ceases, but the cause which produced them is considerably increased; we have then to repair the existing evil, as also that caused by the remedy. If this is not quickly remedied the effect is again produced more speedily than before, and if we are obliged to purge again, the evil is increased a second time; the intestines also become sluggish and hence they do not fulfill their functions; farther they are never evacuated naturally, in a word, purgatives when the primæ viæ in invalids are obstructed, never diminish the effect except by increasing the cause, and never remedy for a time except by augmenting the disease. Hence this method is still too much pursued, it is pleasing to the patients, it seems more prompt, and in fact, provided they are not too much debilitated, they are relieved for a few days; the evil it is true returns, but it is attributed to the insufficiency rather than to the operation of the remedy; further the patients generally wish for present relief, and few physicians have courage to oppose them. It is however important, in medicine as in morals, to sacrifice the present for the future; the neglect of this law peoples the world with unhappy valetudinarians. We wish that we could impress both on physicians and patients, the fine remarks in the mythology of Gaubius, on the bad effects produced by the use of purgatives.

It will be asked, are there not cases where emetics and purgatives may be prescribed the patients mentioned by us? Doubtless there are some, but they are very rare, and we must take care not to be deceived by the signs which seem to indicate purgatives, but which often depend on a cause which must be treated with other remedies. We shall not detail these distinctions here; they would be out of place, we shall merely remark that purgatives ought rarely to be used in this disease. Lewis thinks that a mild emetic may be useful in preparing the primæ viæ for other remedies; but he does not wish more than this from it; several cases have taught me that we may and often should exceed it: and we have mentioned previously two cases of Hoffman, which prove the danger of this remedy. Without experience, good sense alone would convince, that a remedy which causes convulsions is by no means proper in diseases caused by reiterated convulsions.

The evil of the disease is destroyed by combating the cause: by removing it a little each day, we are sure the effect will disappear and not return. If we think only of the effect, the labor of each day is not only useless to the following day, but most generally injurious.

Having mentioned what should be avoided, what must be done? We have stated above the characters which ought to be possessed by the remedies; they should strengthen but not irritate. There are some which can fulfill these two indications but they are few; the two most powerful are undoubtedly cinchona and cold baths. The first remedy independent of its febrifuge virtues, has been considered one of the most powerful tonics, and as soothing. The most celebrated modern physicians consider it as a specific in nervous diseases. We have seen that it was prescribed by Boerhaave, as mentioned above, and Vandermonde used it as stated in the treatment of a young man, who was reduced by excessive sexual intercourse to a very deplorable state. Lewis prefers it to all other remedies, and Stehelin, in the letter mentioned several times, likewise considers it the most efficacious of any.

Twenty years of correct observation have demonstrated, that cold baths possess the same qualities. Dr. Bayard has proved their uses more particularly in diseases produced by onanism; a venereal excess, especially in a case where independent of impotence and simple gonorrhea, there was so much debility, increased it is true by blood-letting and purgatives, that the sick person was considered on the edge of the tomb.

Lewis speaks still more positively of their efficacy: "of all external or internal remedies, there are none equal to the cold baths. They refresh, they strengthen the nerves, and assist transpiration more powerfully than any internal remedy; when well managed, they are more efficacious in dorsal consumption than all other remedies combined." We must even remark that cold baths, as we have already said of the air, are peculiarly advantageous, as their action expends less of the powers of nature than the other remedies: the latter acts only on the vital parts, cold baths give strength even to dead parts.

The union of cinchona and cold baths, is indicated upon the similarity of their powers, they produce the same effects; and being combined, they cure those diseases which other remedies only modify. Tonics, sedatives, and febrifuges, restore the strength, diminish the febrine of the nervous heat, and calm those irregular motions produced by the spasmodic disposition of the nervous system. They remedy debility of the stomach, and very soon relieve the pains which result from it. They restore the appetite, and facilitate digestion and nutrition: they re-establish all the secretions, and especially the transpiration: hence they are so efficacious in all catarrhal and cutaneous diseases, in a word, they remedy all diseases caused by debility, if the patient be not attacked with irremovable obstructions, with inflammation, abcesses, or internal ulcers, which conditions do not necessarily, or almost necessarily, exclude only the cold baths, but often admit the use of cinchona.

We saw some years since, a foreigner, twenty-three or twenty-four years old, who from his earliest youth, had been affected with acute and almost constant pains in the head, which were always attended with loss of appetite. The disease was somewhat lessened by bleeding, evacuations, purgatives, warm baths, broths, and numerous other remedies. I prescribed cold baths and cinchona. The fits daily become less frequent, and weaker. The patient at the end of a month thought himself radically cured; the omission of the remedies, and the bad season renewed the fits, but they were infinitely less violent than before: he again returned to the same course of medicine the following spring. I am persuaded that the same course repeated once or twice, will be attended with a radical cure.

A man, twenty-eight years old, had been affected for some years with an intermittent gout, which always attacked his head, and affected his face very much: he had consulted several physicians, and had tried remedies of various kinds; recently a medicinal wine composed of the most powerful aromatics, infused in Spanish wine had been used; all, and particularly the latter had increased the disease: blisters had been applied to his legs, which occasioned violent symptoms. We were consulted at this period. I advised a strong decoction of cinchona and camomile, which he continued to use for six weeks: this contributed to his health more than any thing he had tried for a number of years. It would be useless to mention a greater number of instances, particularly those foreign to the subjects. To prove the strengthening nature of these remedies, so long demonstrated, and the use of which is indicated in this disease, has been proved by numerous cases.

When I have employed the cinchona in the liquid form, I have ordered a decoction of one ounce of bark, to twelve ounces of water, or according to the indication of red wine, this was allowed to remain for two hours in a close vessel: of this, the dose was three ounces, three times a day.

I order cold baths in the evening, when the dinner is entirely digested; they serve to produce a good night's rest. I know a young man addicted to this habit, whose nights were restless and who was bathed in the morning with colliquative sweats, after the sixth bath he slept five hours and awoke in the morning free from sweats, and much improved.

The preparations of iron are a third remedy, so much employed in all cases of debility, that it is unnecessary to speak of their efficacy as a tonic: as they have no stimulant properties, they are admirably adapted to these diseases: I give them in substance or in a liquid form; but the best preparation is in the natural mineral waters, particularly those of Spa; they are one of the most powerful tonics known, and so far from irritating, removes every thing acrid from the system. Gum myrrh bitters, and the mildest aromatics are also useful. Circumstances must decide on the choice of these medicines. The first mentioned are generally preferred, but some cases may be found which require the others; we may generally select them from the class of those acting on the nerves, using in our choice those precautions mentioned above. It is a disease of the nerves, and must be treated as such, as is often done, and with success without knowing the reason why. It is true, and it has been proved by positive demonstration, that ignorance of this cause, (and hence the neglect of the caution it requires), has sometimes destroyed the effect of apparently the best treatment, although physicians were unable to account for their want of success.

I ordered a young man whose case was mentioned in an extract from his letter, some pills made of myrrh, and a decoction of cinchona, which were very successful. "I perceive every day," he writes, sixteen days after commencing these remedies, "how beneficial they are; the headache is neither so frequent or so violent, and it affects me only when very much fatigued: my stomach is much benefited, and I rarely have pains in my limbs." At the end of a month he was perfectly cured, although perhaps he will never attain his growth. The check in the growth of the machine, is attended with consequences which can never be repaired. May this truth be impressed on the minds of young men. It has for a long time been told them. "Youth," says Linnæus, "is an important time to build up a robust constitution. Nothing is more to be dreaded than the premature or excessive use of venereal pleasures; it causes debility in the sight, vertigo, loss of appetite, and even the debility of the mind. A body enervated in youth, is never restored. Its old age comes soon and life is short." Sixteen hundred years before this great naturalist, Plutarch, in his fine work on the education of children, has recommended the formation of their temperament as extremely important. "No care which contributes to the elegance and strength of the body should be neglected; for," adds he, "the foundation of happy old age is a good constitution in youth; temperance and moderation at this age, are a passport to happiness in the latter years of life."

We may add to this case, the success of which appears owing to the cinchona, another in which cold baths were the principal remedy. A young man of bilious temperament, became addicted to this bad habit at the age of ten years, and had been from that time weak and languid: he had some bilious diseases which were extremely difficult to be cured; and was extremely thin, pale, weak, and sad. I ordered cold baths with a powder of cream of tartar, and a little canella. In less than six weeks he became stronger than he ever was before.

One great advantage of the Spa waters is, that their use causes milk to be digested. The waters of Spa, with some others possess this advantage. We have seen above, that Hoffman ordered asses' milk, mixed with one third of Seltzer water. De la Wettrie has related a successful case of

Boerhaave, "this amiable duke, became impotent; I restored to him his powers by using Spa water with milk."

Debility of the stomach which renders digestion too slow, acrids, inactivity of the bile, and engorgements in the abdominal viscera, are the principal causes which prevent the milk from being digested and which do not permit its use. The waters remedy all these causes, only by assisting digestion; and the cinchona which fulfills the same indications, can also be very well united with the milk. These remedies must be employed either before, to prepare the passages which is generally necessary, or at the same time.

In 1753, I restored to perfect health, a stranger who was so much exhausted, by connection with a courtezan, that he was incapable of an act of virility; his stomach was also extremely enfeebled; and the want of nutrition and sleep had rendered him very thin. At six o'clock in the morning he took six ounces of the decoction of cinchona, with a table spoonful of Canary wine; one hour after he took ten ounces of fresh goat's milk, with a little sugar and an ounce of orange-flower water. He dined on cold roast chicken, bread, and a glass of excellent Burgundy wine with as much water. At six o'clock in the evening he took another dose of cinchona, and at half past six a cold bath, in which he remained ten minutes; he then went to bed. At eight o'clock he took the same quantity of milk, and set up from nine o'clock till ten. Such was the effect of these remedies, that in eight days he cried out with joy on re-entering his chamber, that he had recovered the external mark of virility, to use

Buffon's expression. In one month he had almost entirely regained his primitive strength.

Some absorbent powders, some spoonsful of mint water, and often the addition of a little sugar may also serve to prevent the change in the milk. We may also employ the gum, recently introduced in some parts of England termed the red gum of Gambia, and on which is a small dissertation, in the excellent collection published by the new society of physicians at London; it strengthens and sweetens; these are the two great indications in the diseases of which we are speaking.

Finally, if with all our care it is impossible to retain the milk, we may try butter-milk. I advised it successfully to a young man in whom hypochondriasis made me fearful of common milk. Bilious persons drink it with pleasure and it agrees with them; it should be preferred to milk, whenever there is much heat, a little fever, or an erysipelatous disposition, and is especially very useful, when venereal excesses produce an acute fever of which Raphael died. Notwithstanding the debility, tonics may injure; bleeding is dangerous. The celebrated Johnston, who died baron of Ziebendrof, more than eighty years since, positively forbid it in this case. The cooling treatment is not successful, as Vandermonde has proved and as I have seen; but butter-milk succeeds very well provided it is not too fat. It calms, mitigates, and refreshes; and at the same time nourishes and strengthens; which is very important in this case, where the strength is lost very quickly.

Gilchrist, who does not think much of milk in phthisis, praise butter-milk in the same disease, very much.

Since the last edition of this work, published some years ago, I have been consulted by several enervated persons; some have been entirely cured, and some considerably relieved, while others have gained nothing; when the disease has reached a certain point, we can only hope that its progress will be arrested by remedies. I am ignorant of a part of the results of these cases.

In almost all the cases which have been cured, milk has been the principal food, and cinchona, iron, sulphurous waters, and cold baths the remedies. I have kept some of the patients on a milk diet; others have taken it only twice a day.

The patient whose case is detailed in the sixth section, where I promised to give the treatment, lived for three months on milk, stale bread, one or two fresh eggs, and cold water. He took milk four times a day, twice from the cow without bread, and twice warmed with bread. The remedy was an opiate, composed of cinchona, conserve of orange-peel, and syrup of mint; his stomach was covered with an aromatic plaster, and his whole body was rubbed every morning with flannel; he walked and rode as much as possible, and spent much of his time in the open air. His debility and pains in the chest, prevented the use of cold baths at this period. The success of the remedies was so great, that his strength returned, his stomach regained its powers; and at the end of a month he was able to walk a league; the vomiting ceased entirely, the pains in his chest were very much diminished, and he continued for more than three years in a tolerable state of health; he gradually returned to his usual diet, having become disgusted with milk.

The genital organs always recover their strength the most slowly, and often not at all; although the other parts of the body are perfectly re-established; we may in fact literally say, that the parts which offended first, are those which perish. I have always found it more easy to cure those exhausted by great excesses, when of mature age, than those who have indulged less frequently, but have began in early youth, and have impeded their growth, and have never acquired all their strength. The first may be considered as having had a very violent disease, which has exhausted all their powers: but the organs being perfect, although they have suffered much, they may be re-established by the cause ceasing to act, by time, regimen, and remedies. The temperament of the second has never been formed; how then can it be re-established? It is necessary that art should do in mature age, what nature has been prevented from accomplishing in infancy and youth; but this hope is futile, and observations every day prove, that those young men addicted to this vice in infancy, at the period of puberty, which period is a crisis of nature, and for which all its powers are necessary, observation, I say, proves that these young men must never expect to be vigorous and robust, and they are very fortunate if they enjoy moderate health, free from severe diseases and pains.

Those who repent late, at an age when the machine is preserved, if well regulated, but when it is restored with difficulty, must not have great hopes. When more than forty years old, a man rarely grows young.

When I order cinchona with wine, I do not confine them to milk diet, but I prescribe the remedy in the morning, and the milk at night. I have found some patients for whom it was necessary to change this order; wine taken in the morning always produced vomiting.

When I employ mineral waters, some bottles are drunk pure, before mingling it with milk.

When the disease is inveterate, it usually changes into cacochymia, which must be removed before attempting to re-establish the strength; in this case purgatives are indispensably necessary, and operate very efficaciously. Tonics, nourishment, and milk, if ordered in these cases, produce a slow fever, and the patient loses his strength in proportion as he employs them.

When prompt excesses suddenly cause such debility that the life of the patient is in danger, we must use active cordials, give Spanish wine with a little bread, succulent broths with fresh eggs, put the patient to bed, and apply on the stomach flannels wrung out in hot wine and laudanum.

When venereal excesses have caused an acute fever, bleeding should not be employed, unless indicated by a full and hard pulse; two small bleedings are better than one which is large. Barley-water with a little milk, some nitre, demulcent injections, warm foot-baths, and for nourishment veal broth, are the remedies really indicated, and these have succeeded very promptly in the cases wherein we have employed them.

The symptoms rarely demand a special treatment, but yield to the general treatment. Sometimes however we may employ external in connection with internal tonics, when we wish to strengthen one part in particular; we have often used successfully, fomentations and aromatic plasters to the stomach, and it is also useful to envelope the testicles with fine flannel steeped in some tonic liquid, and to support them with a suspensory bandage.

We may here introduce the remarks of Gotter; "I have sometimes cured gutta serena, occasioned by venereal excesses, by internal tonics, and errhines, which by their slight irritation, cause a greater flow of nervous influence to the optic nerve."

It would be useless to enter more into detail with respect to the cure; however extensive might be our remarks on this subject, it could never guide the patient without the aid of a physician to whom they would be useless. I have treated more fully of the regimen, because when the disease has not progressed far, the removal of the cause, and attention to the regimen, may alone effect a cure, and each one may attend to it without any danger. In order to conclude this part, we have now to mention the prevention. A man well known in the literary world, by his works, and still more respectable for his talents, his knowledge, and his personal qualities, as well as for his name, and the offices which he has filled in one of the first cities of Switzerland, Iselin, secretary of state at Basle, has very politely mentioned this defect of the first edition. I shall quote the fragment of his letter with much more pleasure, as he points out precisely what is necessary to be done. "I wish," said he, "to see from your hand, a work in which you shall explain the surest and least dangerous means, by which parents, while educating their children, and young men, when left to themselves, may avoid those violent desires, which lead to excesses productive of such horrid diseases, or to those disorders which disturb their own happiness and that of society. I am certain that there is a diet peculiarly favorable to continence. I believe that a work which will mention it to us, and will describe the diseases produced by incontinence, would be more valuable than the best moral treatise on this subject."

He is doubtless correct; this addition which he requests is very important, but it is very difficult to separate it from other parts of education not only medicinally but morally. In order to treat upon this subject separately, I must establish a great number of principles, which would extend this small volume too far. Some general precepts, apart from the necessary principles and divisions, would not only be useless, but might become dangerous; thus it is better to defer this treatise, and introduce it in a larger work, on the mode of forming a good constitution, and of imparting to young men firm health; which subject although treated by able men, is not yet exhausted, and to which may be added a number of very important things, as also on the diseases of this age; we shall not therefore treat upon this subject here. All that we can say is, that laziness, inactivity, lying too long in bed, a soft bed, a succulent diet, spices, salt, wine, and licentious books, are the causes most proper to produce these excesses, and hence they cannot be too carefully avoided. Diet is very important and is not sufficiently attended to. Those who educate young men, should have before them the fine remarks of St. Jerome. "The forge of Vulcan, the volcanoes of Vesuvius, and of mount Olympus, do not burn more than those young men who live upon succulent meats, and indulge in wine." Menjot, one of the physicians of Louis the Great, from the middle to the end of the last age, mentions females in whom venereal ecstacy was caused by an excess.

The use of wine and meat is much more detrimental inasmuch as while wine increases the excitement of the body, it diminishes the strength of mind which must resist it. "Wine and meat, blunt the soul," says Plutarch in his treatise on meats, which deserves an extensive circulation. The most ancient physicians were well acquainted with the effect of regimen on the manners: they had the idea of a moral medicine, and Galen has left us a small work on this subject, which is now the best treatise extant. One will be convinced after reading it of the reality of his promise. "That those who deny that the difference in food, renders some temperate and others dissolute; some chaste, others incontinent; some courageous and others cowardly; some mild and others quarrelsome; some modest, others presumptuous: let those, I say, who deny this truth come to me; let them follow my directions in regard to eating and drinking, and I will promise them, that their moral philosophy shall be very much improved; they will percieve the powers of their mind augmented, they will acquire more genius, more memory, more prudence, and more diligence.

I will tell them also, what drinks, what winds, what temperature, or countries they must avoid or select." Hippocrates, Plato, Aristotle and Plutarch had already left some very good remarks on this important subject; and among the works of the Pythagorean Porphyrius, the Pagan zealot of the third century, there is one on the abstinence from meats, in which he reproaches Firmus Castricius for having left the vegetable diet, although he had asserted it was the most proper for preserving health, and for facilitating the study of philosophy, and adds, "since you have eaten meat, your experience has taught you, that this statement was well founded." There are some very good remarks in this work.

The most efficacious preservative, and in fact the only infallible one, is that mentioned by that great man who best knew his equals and all their ways: who saw not only what they are, but what they have been, what they should be and what they might become; who has most truly loved them, who has made the greatest efforts in their favor, who has sacrificed himself for them, and who has been most cruelly persecuted. "Watch carefully over this young man, leave him alone neither day nor night, at least sleep in his chamber. When he has contracted this habit, the most fatal to which a young man can be subject, he will carry its baneful effects with him to the tomb, his mind and body will be always enervated." I refer to the work itself for the other excellent remarks on this subject.

A description of the danger, when one is addicted to this vice, is perhaps the most powerful motive for arresting it. It is a frightful picture, and makes one shudder. Let us mention its principal characters. A general wasting of the animal machine, a debility of all the bodily senses, and of all the faculties of the mind: the loss of the imagination, and of the memory: imbecility, the shame and the disgrace attendant upon it, all the functions disturbed, suspended, or painful, long, severe, and disgusting diseases, the pain sharper and constantly recurring: all the diseases of old age in the period of vigor: an inaptitude for all the occupations for which man was born, the humiliating thought of being only a useless weight on the earth, the mortifications to which he is daily exposed: the disgust for all honorable pleasures; weariness, an aversion for others and for himself; horror of life, and the dread of some day committing suicide, anguish of mind worse than the pains, and remorse worse than the anguish, which increases daily, and doubtless assumes new power, when the soul is enfeebled only by attachment to the body, will serve perhaps for eternal punishment, and unquenchable fire. This is a sketch of the fate reserved for those, who act as if they did not fear it.

Before leaving the subject of treatment, I will mention to patients, (and this remark applies also to all those affected with chronic diseases, especially when attended with debility), that they must not think in a few days to repair the evils which are caused by the errors of years. They must expect to be a long time under treatment, and to confine themselves strictly to the rules of regimen; and if they sometimes appear minute, it is because they are not in a state to perceive their importance; and they must constantly remember, that the tediousness of the strictest cure is much less than that of the slightest disease. I will take the liberty of remarking, that if some diseases which are curable are not cured from malpractice; there are a great many which are not cured from the indocility of the patient, notwithstanding the best of medical advice. Hippocrates required, in order to insure himself success, that the patient, the physician, and assistant should do their duty: if this concurrence were less rare, happy results would be more frequent. "Let the patient," says Aretæus, "be brave, and conspire with the physician against the disease." I have seen the most obstinate maladies yield to this harmony of action; and very recent observations have demonstrated, that even cancerous diseases have yielded to remedies prescribed, perhaps with some skill, but employed with a docility and regularity, eulogized by their successes.

ARTICLE IV.

ANALOGOUS DISEASES.

SECTION XI.

NOCTURNAL POLLUTANTS.

I have mentioned the dangers of too great an evacuation of semen from venereal excesses and onanism; and I have said at the commencement of the work, it was discharged also in nocturnal pollutions, by lascivious dreams, and by a discharge termed simple gonorrhea. I shall briefly examine these two diseases.

The mind is united to the body by such laws, that even when the senses are enchained by sleep, it is occupied by ideas which has been presented to it during the day.

> Lex quæ in vita usurpant homines, cogitant, curant, vident
> Quæque aiunt vigilantes agitantque, ea si cui in somno accidunt,
> Minus, mirum est.
>
> —Acc.

Another law of this union is, that without distributing the other senses, without rendering them sensible to external impressions; the soul may excite the motions necessary to execute the wishes suggested by the ideas which exist in it. Engrossed in ideas of the pleasures of love, addicted to lascivious dreams, the objects pictured by it produce on the genital organs the same motions as if awake, and the act is physically consummated, if it only be imagined. We know what occurred to Horace on his journey to Brindes.

> Hic ego mendacem stultissimis usque puellam
> Ad mediam noctem expecto: somnus tamen aufert
> Intentum veneri: turn immundo somnia visu
> Nocturnam vestem maculant ventremque supinum.

These organs in turn irritated first, sometimes excite the imagination, and cause dreams which terminate like the preceding.

These principles serve to explain the different kind of pollutions.

The first comes from an excess of semen, and it occurs in powerful young men, who are sanguinary, strong, and chaste. The warmth of the bed rarifies the fluids, and the semen being more capable of rarefaction than any other, the irritated vesicles affect the imagination, which deprived of the aids which delude it, is entirely devoted to it; the idea of coition produces the last effect, emission. In this case this evacuation is not a disease, but rather a favorable crisis, a motion which procured the discharge of a fluid, which, if too abundant and retained too long, might be injurious: and although several physicians, who believe only what they see, do not deny but that this fluid may, by its abundance, produce diseases different from priapism or furor uterinus.

May I be allowed here a short digression on this question, it is not foreign to the subject.

"A semine retento multos produci morbos memorat Galenus, et exemplum in historia monstrat. Ille novit virum et mulierem quibus hujusmodi erat natura, qui præ viduitate a lubidinis usu abstinentes, torpidi pigrique facti sunt. Homo cibi cupiditatem amisit, atque ne exiguam quidem ciborum partem concoquere potuit: ubi vero se ipsum cogendo, plus cibi ingerebat, protinus ad vomitum excitabatur: mœstus etiam apparebat, non solum has ob causas, sed etiam (ut melancholici solent) citra manifestam occasionem; mulier vero, præter cœtera mala, nervorum quoque distentione vexabatur. Verum hi quam celerrime liberati sunt, ad pristinam consuetudinem reversi. Dum Montis Pessulani eram, observationem fere per similem vidi. Mulier valens, quadragesimum ætatis suæ; annum complens, exiguo post tempore vidua; quæ antea cum viri concubitu gauderet hoc omnino post obitum ejus fuerit privata, incidit tam violenter in affectu histerico, ut dificere videretur actiones sensuum: cum nullum remedium in ea accessus tolerare potuerat, nisi titillatio partium genitalium (veluti per coïtum usu venire solet). Inde agitabatur toto corpore, et a copiosa pollutione seminis evacuabatur; quo facto libera est mulier a molestia sua."

"Aliam observationem Zacutus refert; exeadem causa patiebatur puella quæ ex intervallis paroxysmo ita convellebatur; ut accedente difficili respiratione, tota convulsa, sine sensu ullo, oculis distortis, nimio dentium stridore præedente cum lingua tremula, animam efflare videretur. Cui cum plurima auxilia quæ in hac occasione utilia sunt, non juvarent, pessaria ex acri confecta utero applicanda curavit. ex quorum admotione, titillatione et fervore quodam in utero concitato, copiosum semen excernens, ab accessione sæva superstes remansit."

"Historiam monialis Hoffmannus enarrat, quæ ob eamdem causam, ab eadem evacuatione, aliquoties paroxysmum solvebat."

Homines duo, inquit Zacutus, quum concubitu quo antea creberrime utebantur, privarentur, in gravissima damna incurrere: alter in otio et mollitie educatus cum tabi esset propinquus, a coïtu cum cessarit, huic sensim, et sine sensu umbilicus intumuit. Nuptus, et ad concubitum reversus, sanitatem recuperavit. Alter vero nobillissimus, adeo erat coïtus studio deditus, ut lassatus et debilis cogeretur hac de causa ad tempus lecto quiescere. Ecce post sex menses, nausea correptus, vertigine concutitur, et post paucos dies epilepsia sæva opprimitur. Ab accessione auxiliorum ope levatus, medicorum præsidia expostulat. Hi, sympathicam epilepsiam a vitio ventiiculi subortam rati, tonum et ventriculum a vitiosis humoribus expurgant, et roborant, sed frustra. Nam malo ferocius infestante, post paucas horas velut sideratus extinctus est. Dissecto corpore, nullum vitium in stomacho, cerebro, reliquisque partibus inventum, præterquam in cavitate vasis semen in penem deferentis et ulceribus sordidis, ab hac virulenta substantia retenta concretis."

"Dom. Zinde dissertationem Bassileæ publicavit, jam quindecim ab hinc annis, ubi observationes morborum a semine retento acri productis in unum colligit, quæ lectu non indignæ sunt."

"Hic subjici potest quæ Dom. Sauvages dixit, de mulierum castitate; quæ pudori litant, sed tanta veneris cupiditate incenduntur, et eo ardentius ac miserabilius flagrat, quo ardorem suum regunt accuratius: inde mœror, agrypnia, anorexia, macies, pollutiones frequentes. Ille celebris medicus puellam novit hujuscemodi quæ ad senis putidi et inficeti pedes prostata et acerrime suam calamitatem deplorans, interea hisco invitis seminis profluviis erat obnoxia a duobus annis his miseriis cruciata, et castimoniam mentis intemeratam servans: immane patiebatur veneris desiderium sensitivum cui constanter reluctabatur voluntas."

A physician respectable for his knowledge and age, who has long followed the Austrian armies in Italy, states that he has observed that those German soldiers who were not married and were chaste, were often affected with epilepsy, priapisms, or nocturnal pollutions, which supervene from the semen, which is perhaps also more acrid in a climate warmer than their own, and where the diet is more succulent.

Dr. Jacques whom we have already quoted, had written a treatise on the diseases produced by avoiding venereal pleasures. Reneaume has written another on virginity which has the same object.

Finally, to omit some others, Gaubius mentions excessive continence among the causes of the disease. "It rarely," says he, "produces some evils. In some men however, who have a sanguineous temperament, and in whom the secretion of semen is very abundant, and in some females; we ought not then to deny its existence, but we may assert its rarity, especially in this age, which seems one of debility: and we are deceived every day, if we attribute indirectly to this cause, all the diseases which attack unmarried people, by recommending marriage as a remedy: which is often badly indicated, and which is frequently injurious, because it cannot destroy the vices which attend the disease, and we must not add to those bad symptoms which have passed those generally produced in languid persons by pregnancy and parturition. We return to the pollutions.

It has been seen that the first kind, is produced by a superabundance of semen, which evacuated, is not bad in itself; but may become so by recurring too frequently, even when the excess is not injurious. We have already remarked that one evacuation disposes to another, so great is the force of habit, which is facilitated by certain feelings, and they are produced by the slightest cause: a useful remark on the intelligence of the animal economy, on which Galen, and particularly Maty, have made excellent remarks, but which however has not been fully treated of; this inconvenience results from it, that it is followed by unnecessary evacuations. They are then very injurious, and are attended with all the dangers of excessive evacuations produced in other modes. Satyrus, surnamed Grypalopex, who resided at Thasus, had from the age of twenty-five, frequent nocturnal pollutions; he died of consumption when thirty years old.

Zimmermann mentions a man of fine talent, who had lost all the activity of his mind, and whose body was in the state described by Boerhaave. We have seen the ill consequences observed by Hoffman follow pollutions. The most common symptoms when the disease has not made great progress, are a constant exhaustion, which is greater in the morning, and acute pains in the kidneys. Some months since I was consulted by a vine-dresser, about fifty years old, who, although robust, was so much exhausted by excessive discharges, that he could only work a few hours each day, and was often confined to his bed by pains in the kidneys, and constantly became thinner. I gave him some advice, but am unacquainted with the results.

I knew a man who became deaf after a cold which was neglected, and who was more deaf whenever he had an emission, which was also attended with indisposition; and another enfeebled by various causes, who after a nocturnal emission, awoke in such a general state of stupidity, that he remained as it were paralysed, for half an hour, and was debilitated for twenty-four hours after.

We may mention in the first class, the pollutions of those who having had frequent emissions, suddenly suspend them: this was the case with a widow-woman mentioned by Galen; she had been a widow for a long time, and the retention of the semen, caused a disease of the uterus; in sleep she had convulsive motions in her loins, arms, and legs, which were attended with an abundant discharge of thick semen, with the same sensation as in coition.

A dancer was accidentally wounded near the left breast; the surgeon prescribed a strict diet, and forbade her the pleasures she often enjoyed. The third night after this privation, to which she submitted, but neglected the diet, she had an emission, which returning several times the succeeding nights, she became very thin, and was affected with severe pains in the kidneys. The wound continued to heal, and would have been cured, provided her food and drink had been regulated. The surgeon, firm in his principles, continued his prohibition, and resorted to bleeding and purgatives. Exhausted and enfeebled, she omitted the remedies and resumed her old habits; debility and pains soon disappeared.

But beware of concluding from this case, that the precepts of the greatest surgeons are useless, which being founded on other observations, strictly interdict coition to those wounded: every practitioner can judge for himself how injurious it is. I will mention an instance where masturbation was fatal, and which has been mentioned by Fabricius of Hilden. Cosmers Sotan had amputated a young man's hand, which had been injured by a gun; as he knew him to be very ardent, he prohibited his indulgence with his wife, when also he warned him of the danger. But when all the symptoms were relieved, and the cure was progressing, the patient feeling desires to which his wife not respond, he had an emission of semen without coition, which was immediately followed with fever, delirium, convulsions, and other violent symptoms, which caused death in four hours.

I have seen a young married man, who, on jumping from a chaise, fell on his side, the wheel passed over his foot, between the heal and instep; there was no fracture nor dislocation, but a severe contusion; recovering in five days, his conduct was the same as if there, had been no accident;

two hours after the whole leg was inflamed with very severe pains, and violent fever, which continued nearly thirty hours. Our remarks at the beginning of this section, on the connection between dreams, and the ideas presented to the mind during the day, serve to explain why those addicted to onanism, are so subject to nocturnal emissions; their minds occupied the whole day with venereal ideas, picture the same objects at night, and the lascivious dreams are followed by an evacuation, which will always take place readily, when the organs are by any means irritable.

It is important to forewarn one early of the progress of this habit; and whatever may be the first cause of the pollutions, not to allow them to be inveterate; when they have continued a long time they are difficult to cure. "There is no disease," says Hoffman, "so troublesome to the patients and physicians as nocturnal emissions, which are of long continuance, and which have become habitual, particularly when they return daily." The best remedies are often useless, and frequently do more harm than good.

Every physician who has written on this disorder, states that the cure is very difficult, and all physicians who have had occasion to treat it, have themselves experienced it. Unless the powers of the organs can be restored, or their irritability between the time of two pollutions can be diminished, or the return of lascivious dreams can be suddenly prevented, which is not more easy, we may be sure that the emissions will return, and nearly destroy all the good caused by the small quantity of remedies employed since the last; we then can gain but very little between two pollutions, and hence a long time is necessary before a sensible effect is produced.

Cœlius Aurelianus has collected the best remarks of the ancients on the treatment. He enjoins 1st, That the patient should avoid as much as possible, all objects of desire. 2d., That he should sleep upon a hard and refreshing bed; that a thin plate of lead should be applied to the kidneys: that sponges dipped in water and vinegar, or in cold lotions should be applied to the genital parts. 3d., That he should use only food and drinks which refresh; he recommends, 4th., Tonics. 5th., The use of the cold bath. 6th., Never to lay on the back, but always on the side or belly. His advice is very good, but let us see more distinctly what is the indication: it is to diminish the quantity of the semen, and to prevent the dreams.

This is fulfilled much better by the diet and general regimen than by remedies. The most proper food is vegetables and fruits: and among the meats those which contain the least substance; in both classes those must be chosen which are not acrid. We have already seen above, the influence of this regimen on the tranquility of the sleep, and it cannot be too much recommended to persons affected with nocturnal pollutions, to whom this diet is necessary. They should avoid suppers particularly, or at least should eat but lightly; attention to this alone, will contribute more to the cure than any other remedy.

Some years since, I saw a young man who was affected with nocturnal emissions almost every night; and who already had some attacks of nightmare. A surgeon barber ordered him to drink while lying down some glasses of warm water, which did not diminish the emissions, but increased the last disease; the two diseases united and returned every night: the phantom of the nightmare was a female, which caused at the same time the emission. Enfeebled by these two causes, by the loss of tranquil sleep, he was rapidly advancing into consumption.

I ordered him to taste only for supper a little bread, and some ripe fruit; to sup early and to take on getting into bed, a glass of cold water with fifteen drops of Hoffman's anodyne mixture. He was soon able to sleep quietly, the two diseases disappeared entirely, and he regained his strength.

Indigestible and dark meats, especially in the evening, are a real poison in this disease; and I repeat it, without the privation of supper, other remedies are useless. Wine, liquors, and coffee are injurious in several ways. The best drink is pure water, in each bottle of which a drachm of nitre may be successfully dissolved; a short time since, however, a patient was injured by nitre, which caused emissions more frequently; I attributed this effect to two causes: one, because his nerves were very weak, and in such a temperament, the nitre acts as an irritant; the other, is that it increases the quantity of urine; the bladder is filled more quickly at night, and we know the fulness of the bladder is one of the causes of emissions.

The precepts of Coelius to avoid soft beds is of the utmost importance: feather beds should be avoided, and straw is better than hair; I have seen some patients who slept upon leather. The advice not to lay upon the back is also necessary; this posture is injurious, as the sleep is more disturbed by keeping the genital organs warm. Finally, as habit has here a great effect, and as it is important to break it, the following observation may furnish one means of success. I have it from an Italian, who is respectable for his virtues, and one of the most excellent men I have ever seen. He consulted me for a very different disease; but in order to instruct me better, he gave me the whole history of his health; he had been incommoded by frequent emissions, which entirely exhausted him. He resolved strongly in the evening to awake the first moment a female appeared to his imagination, and was occupied with this idea for a long time before sleeping. The remedy was very successful, the idea of danger, and the wish to awake intimately united with the idea of time at this latter; he awoke in time, and the precaution repeated several nights removed the evil.

But the last two cases inspire too much. security; there are some which cannot be remedied; that mentioned by Hoffman is an instance, and we ought to advise the patient, that it is useless to expect any advantage without persevering in the use of remedies. A long time is necessary, as in this case, where regimen is essential, an evident benefit cannot be expected unless it is pursued for several weeks. If these remedies are employed, they should be founded on the same indication as the regimen. Not long since we saw disease produced by a large bleeding: powders of nitre, lemonade, acids, and orgeat may be useful.

Hoffman employed in one addicted to onanism, who, on leaving off the practice, was effected with emissions, the following powder.

R. C. C. pphice. ppat.
Ossis sepiæ aa. . . . . oz. ss.
Succini cum instillat olei tart. per deliqueum ppat. dr. ij.
Carb. cal. . . . . dr. i.

One drachm of this should be taken at night with black cherry water; in the morning Seltzer water and milk: for drink, a ptisan of cichory or canella. By this medicine and by proper diet, the sick person was cured in a few weeks. Zimmermann also has cured by the same powder, a case in which there were very frequent pollutions, followed by the common gonorrrhea which had existed several years in a young man twenty-one years old. It is difficult to explain the good effects of this powder, which is an absorbent; I have derived the same benefit from camphor.

Another kind of pollution exist in those affected with hypochondriasis. With them the circulation is slow, particularly in the abdominal veins: hence, the parts from which they return the blood are often congested: the nerves are easily excited, their fluids are acrid, and hence are very much disposed to irritate: their sleep is generally disturbed by dreams; hence emissions occur, to which they are extremely subject. Imagination, says Boerhaave, often produces during sleep emissions of semen. The most devoted students are disposed to severe erections, and since the last edition of this work, Thiery, one of the most distinguished physicians in France, has been affected with them.

We may mention here, as consequences of this last kind of pollutions, and attacking principally those addicted to melancholy, a disease which may be called furor genitalis: it differs from priapism, and from satyriasis: the following case will give an idea of it. A man fifty years of age had been affected with it, for more than twenty four years, and in this long time, he had connection with females once in twenty-four hours, or had indulged in onanism, and these acts were generally repeated several times during the day. The semen was clear, acrid, and sterile, and the evacuation was very sudden. His nervous system was excessively enfeebled, the fits of melancholy were frequent, the powers of his mind were enfeebled; his hearing was dulled, his sight extremely weak; he died miserable. I advised no remedies; he had already taken a great number; several of them were useless, and all those which were warm were injurious: cinchona which had been prescribed by Albinus, and which had been taken infused in wine, had proved beneficial, and the authority of this distinguished physician, is a new one in favor of this remedy: among the consultations, is a case nearly similar. The *furor genitalis*, was almost constant, and both mind and body were enfeebled.

SECTION XI.

SIMPLE GONORRHEA.

"GONORRHEA," says Galen who was acquainted only with the simple, "is a running of semen without erection." Several authors in every age, and even Moses speak of it: among the cases of Hippocrates, is one of a mountaineer, in whom the disease seems to have been a gonorrhea, and who had an involuntary discharge of urine and semen. Boerhaave however seems to mention this disease as doubtful. "We read," says he, "in some medical books, that the semen is sometimes discharged imperceptibly, but this disease must be very rare, and we do not know of a case of an emission of semen without some excitement, where real semen secreted in the testicles, and accumulated in the seminal vesicles, was emitted. The fluid of the prostate glands however, is sometimes emitted." This authority is doubtless very respectable: but although Boerhaave does not decide positively, he is opposed by all physicians, and even by some of his own school. Gaubius, one of his most distinguished pupils, admits the imperceptible evacuation of semen. My own observations confirm the existence of both diseases. I have seen men in whom, after an excessive diarrhea, after venereal excesses or onanism, there was a constant running from the penis, but which did not render them incapable of having erections and emissions. They complain even that one emission produces more debility than a running of several weeks; which evidently proves that the liquid of these evacuations, was not the same, and that the fluid of gonorrhea comes from the prostate glands, and from some other glands which surround the urethra, from the follicles, existing in its whole length, or finally; from the dilated exhalent vessels. I have seen others who had, like the former, a running which enfeebled them much more, and rendered them incapable of venereal excitement, of all erection, and hence of all emission; although the testicles seemed to fulfill their functions. It appeared to me demonstrated, that in these latter, the real semen escaped imperceptibly. And when the structure of the genital organs is considered, one is easily persuaded that the first disease is more frequent than the last: but the existence of the latter can be easily understood. Correct authors have termed it real gonorrhea, when the running was real semen, and the other bastard or catarrhal gonorrhea.

The dangers of this running are very great. We have mentioned before, Aretæus' description of it. "How can one be otherwise than weak," says he, "when the strength of life is constantly discharged? It is the semen alone which renders a man strong." Celsus who lived before Aretærus, states positively that the emission of semen without venereal excitement leads to consumption. "John, son of Zechariah, better known as Actuarius, in his work in favor of the ambassador sent by the emperor of Constantinople into the north, thinks like all the authors already mentioned by us." If the discharge of semen without erection and without perceptions continues for some time, it necessarily produces consumption and death, because the most elaborate parts of the fluids and the animal energies are dissipated.

The most modern authors think like the ancients. "The whole body, particularly the back," says Senac, "wastes; the patients become feeble, dry, and pale; they languish, they have pains in the kidneys, they are hollow eyed." Boerhaave arranges this gonorrhea among the causes of paralysis and it may be remarked that in this place he admits gonorrhoea of real semen. "Paralysis," says he, "from gonorrhea is incurable; because the body is exhausted by it." In a fine dissertation of Koempf, are some very interesting cases.

This disease may depend on several remote causes. The proximate cause is commonly combined with a defect in the liquids which escape, which are too limpid and often too acrid, and with a great relaxation in the parts. The defect in the fluids denotes a want of elaboration which depends on general debility: this requires tonics which are indicated by the debility of the organs; concurring circumstances decide on the selection of them. It would be out of place to enter here into all these details on which we find good remarks in several authors and particularly in Sennert, the author of the best abridgement of practical medicine we have.

The same remedies indicated in the course of this work against the other consequences of pollution are useful against this; cold baths, cinchona, preparations of iron, and other tonics. Boerhaave, says hepatica produces excellent effects in inveterate gonorrhea when dependent on relaxation of the organs. Sometimes in order to destroy the tendency of fluids to flow toward the same part, as produced by habit, we may begin by some laxatives. Some celebrated practitioners have ever attributed to them an almost specific efficacy against this disease; experience, still more than reason has proved the contrary to me, and those who will take the trouble of reading the work mentioned above will see that they order no laxatives.

Actuarius prescribes tonics which are not stimulant.

Aretæus thinks it should be remedied immediately, on account of its imminent danger; and orders only tonics, continence, and cold baths.

Celsus, from whose works both have profitted, prescribes frictions, and very cold baths; whatever is eaten must be taken cold, all food which may cause crudities and wind, and increase the acridity of the semen must be avoided. Fernel orders succulent food which is easily digested and tonic electuaries.

If Languius' statement, who asserted that purgatives and diet would cure the disease, be true, it is perhaps only in cases where it is produced by a bad diet, which might have caused obstructions in the abdomen, and vitiated all the fluids, although the solids might not have been affected so severely, and he has seen only this instance of it: for if the attack had been more powerful, the purgatives would necessarily have been aided by tonics. Such was the gonorrhea observed by Regis, and detailed by Craanem. "A man," says he "of a phlegmatic temperament, having used moist food for a long time, was attacked with a running of a vitious aqueous humor, which escaped imperceptibly. He grew thin; his eyes were hollowed, and every day his strength declined." Regis commenced with cathartics to evacuate these pituitary fluids; he then ordered tonics, and dry food: and finally, if this was not sufficient, an issue in each leg. But this treatment by cathartics is never proper, when this disease is the consequence of venereal excesses, and when it depends, as Senac states, on the debility in the seminal vesicles, by being successively in a state of repletion and inactivity so frequently.

Timeus mentions a case which will be in place here. "A young man," says he, "a law student, of a sanguineous temperament, practised masturbation two or three times a day, and sometimes more frequently—he became affected with gonorrhea, attended with general bodily debility. I considered the gonorrhea as a consequence of the relaxation in the seminal vessels, and the debility as dependent on the frequent emission of semen, which had dissipated the natural heat, collected the crudities, injured the nervous system, affected the mind, and debilitated the whole body." He ordered a tonic wine, with astringents and aromatics infused in red wine, an opiate of the same character, and an ointment composed of oil of roses, mastich, nitre, Bol. armenian, fullers-earth, and white wax. The patient was cured of this shameful disease in a month, and I advised him to abstain from this horrid vice, and to think of the Eternal's threat, who excludes all such from the Kingdom of Heaven.[42]

One of the most distinguished physicians in Switzerland, says Zimmermann, G. M. Wepfer of Schaffhousen, whose authority is very great, states that he has cured one person of a constant running caused by masturbation, by a preparation of iron. Veslin of Zurzach confirms this by his experience, and adds my friends have also seen good effects from it.

Professor Stehelin mentions a literary man, who was affected with an involuntary discharge of semen, without any venereal ideas; this was cured by using iron with wine and cinchona. But the same remedies, and also the mineral waters of Swalbac and dashing cold water on the pubis and perineum, were not so successful in a young man in whom this was caused by masturbation. He adds that Dr. Bongars, a celebrated practitioner of Maseyck, has cured two persons affected with debility of the seminal vesicles, by prescribing three times a day, for eight days, ten drops of laudanum, in a glass of Pontac wine, and a decoction of Sarsaparilla. Stehelin remarks that although opium is contra indicated, it has been advised by Etmuller as a remedy for a too prompt emission of semen, dependent upon its being too stimulant. I will add that on examining attentively the advice of this celebrated practitioner, and comparing the nature of the disease in some cases, with the effects of opium, we can easily concieve that this remedy may sometimes be useful, but not in the cases where he advises it. He distinguishes very carefully the different kinds of discharges and mentions the causes and treatment of each, and then passing to the emission which supervenes at the commencement of the erection nimis citam, he mentions two causes of it. 1st., The relaxation of the seminal vesicles. 2d., Too abundant and too fervid semen, in this case he prescribes opium. But for what reason? Opium whose aphrodisiac virtue is so well known; a virtue mentioned by Etmuller in his small work on this remedy, and even where he recommends it, can only increase the cause of the disease, and hence aggravate the symptoms. The cases where it is useful are on the contrary, when the fluids are thin and watery, and the nerves very irritable. We know that it remedies these symptoms, that it suspends the irritability, and that it checks all evacuations except transpiration—but we must repeat that it must be used with care, otherwise it would be injurious. Tralles in his excellent work on this remedy, has mentioned one case, and similar ones may be found in other books, which ought to render us more careful. "A man," says he "who from his youth had been addicted to masturbation, which had rendered him very feeble, never took opium for a cough diarrhea, or for any other purpose, without having during the night lascivious dreams, attended with an emission of semen, which was very injurious." May I be permitted here to make one remark, which naturally presents itself: the error of Etmuller proves very evidently, 1st., How much influence an exact theory has upon practice, which without its aid can only be false and erroneous. 2d., Hence, how much advantage a man possessing both, has over him who is guided by a few cases only, or who is devoted to a system: finally, 3d., How much the perusal of the best practical authors who have denied this correct theory, which must be ascribed to our age, may decieve those who on reasoning believe them implicitly, and who are ignorant of the principles which serve as a touchstone, to distinguish in medicine the good from the bad.

I shall conclude by two of my cases; more would be unnecessary.

A young man twenty years old, who had the misfortune to indulge in onanism, was affected for two months, with a constant discharge of mucus, and nocturnal pollutions, accompanied at times with considerable exhaustion; he had frequent and violent pains in the stomach; his lungs was very feeble, and he perspired easily; I prescribed the following opiate:

R. Conditi rosar. rubr. . . . . oz. iii.
Condit anthos.
Cort Peruv. . . . . a, a, oz. i.
Mastices. . . . . dr. ii.
Olei cinamoni. . . . . gts. iii.
Sirup Cort. Aur. . . . . q. s.
f. electuar. solid

He took a quarter of an ounce of this twice a day. In three weeks he was nearly well; the running ceased, except after the emissions; he continued the same remedy for fifteen days, and then was entirely cured.

A man and his wife, foreigners and strangers, were attacked nearly at the same time, and were certain that they had contracted no disease; there was a running attended with debility and feebleness, along the whole dorsal spine; which evidently proceeded from conjugal excesses; the running was much greater in the husband. They had used various remedies, and among others mercurial pills, which increased the discharge. They consulted me. I prescribed cold baths, and wine, with cinchona, steel, and red roses. They used the remedy regularly: it was in the summer of 1758: the continual rains rendered the use of river baths very difficult; the female used them but two or three times, and the male twelve times in five weeks; they were nearly cured. I ordered them to continue the remedies a short time longer, and they became perfectly well.

This success cannot serve as a foundation for a generally favorable prognosis. I shall mention only one case in support of this opinion, which however can be demonstrated satisfactorily. One of the most celebrated practitioners now in Europe, who has contributed much to the science of medicine; has been affected for more than fifteen years, with a simple gonorrhea, which has resisted his own skill, and that of some other physicians whom he had consulted; this sad disease is gradually wasting his health, and he probably will die long before this would have occurred, in the natural course of events.

It would be useless to say more. I have neglected nothing to awaken the minds of young men, to the horrors of the abyss into which they are plunging. I have pointed out the most proper remedies for the diseases which they bring upon themselves. I shall conclude by repeating what I have already mentioned in the course of the work, that a few fortunate cures must not decieve them; the person most successfully treated, with difficulty regains his former vigor, which is never preserved but by extreme care: the number of those who remain languid, is ten times greater than that of those cured—we should not consider those who have been affected but slightly, or who have been enabled by a more vigorous temperament, as fair examples of the cases.

> Non bene ripæ creditur
> Ipse aries etiam nunc vellera siccat.

APPENDIX.

BY A PHYSICIAN,
Member of the Medical Society of the city
and county of New York.

—

The genital organs of both sexes are somewhat numerous and complicated, and their diseases are not less so; yet it is a melancholy fact, that the greater part of them are produced by a perversion of their functions from their legitimate use. The chief[43] design of these organs is reproduction. Their organization is such, when perfect, as to excite in the individual, desires which are calculated to secure this great end, the perpetuity of the species.

Reproduction is an extension of creation, generally, in definite forms, and is one of the most mysterious and stupendous powers in nature, but one which has been preserved in the organization of all living bodies. This is one of the most admirable conformations bestowed upon animate creation, and happily illustrates the wisdom of that Being who conceived it; for were this organization otherwise, all bodies possessing vitality must soon return to their elementary principles without others to succeed them; and the earth which now contains innumerable inhabitants, and numberless plants, which variegate and beautify, its surface, would become a solitary and barren waste; unless a succession of creations were to follow, which would be in opposition to what we know of the laws which govern the world. Is this power derived from the specific formation of these organs? Or is it from a source independent of this particular organization, although this is necessary inasmuch as it is the only medium through which it can act to this end? The affirmative of the first question is a position sometimes assumed, and contemplates only secondary causes, vitality being considered a consequence of organization. I know of nothing that will countervail the affirmative of the latter, which has in view both primary and secondary causes. We have received from the hands of the Author of Nature, a certain definite formation in the aggregate, this aggregate is compounded of numerous organs, each of which receives a specific organization adapted to the particular function it is destined to perform; this is in conformity to the inflexible and unalterable laws of animal formation; in like manner vitality is imparted as the moving power of the whole machinery. Not that vitality is the product of organization, but that this principal puts in motion inanimate matter and extends itself in definite forms by successive developments. It is obvious that the moving power unaided cannot produce a contrariety of effects, but when acting on organs of different structure, may produce results as diversified as the organs themselves. Hence it is that the liver secretes bile, the kidneys urine, the testicles semen, arid all the other various functions of the body, harmonize together in order to secure the preservation of the individual, and the perpetuity of the species. This is when every function is kept in subordination to its legitimate end. When there is a perversion of uses, the harmony of action is disturbed, not only in the immediate organ affected, but by a law of the animal economy, which we term sympathy, the whole system suffers. This intimate relation between the several functions of the body, is badly represented by the term sympathy. The truth is, the healthy and perfect action of each organ, depends upon that of every other, and this too in the ratio of their dependence. This being the case, one organ does not become diseased without affecting others. The sympathy of the genital system with other parts is very great, hence the disastrous consequences arising from diseases produced by an excessive venereal indulgence, but more particularly by onanism. That this latter practice produces morbid effects on the mind, as well as on the body, may easily be shown. That justly celebrated philosopher and good man, Dr. Rush, in his treatise on the diseases of the mind, says, "four cases of madness occurred in my practice, from *onanism*, between the years of 1804, and 1807. It is induced more frequently by this cause in young men than is commonly supposed by parents and physicians. The morbid effects of intemperance in a sexual intercourse with women, are feeble, and of a transient nature, compared with the train of physical and moral evils which this solitary vice fixes upon the body and mind."

Dr. Eberle, in his *Treatise on the Practice of Medicine*[44] has given an etiological table from which, he makes the following deductions. "It would appear," says he, "that in Paris, insanity from this cause occurs in the proportion of one out of fifty-eight in woman of the lower order of society; and one out of fifty-one in males of the same class. In the higher classes it occurs in both sexes in the ratio of about one to twenty-three." He also enumerates it among the causes of *idiotism*, and, on the authority of Zimmerman, of epilepsy.

"Masturbation," says Esquirol, "this scourge of the human race, is more frequently than is imagined, the cause of *insanity*, particularly among the rich." Here is undoubted authority and the higher classes of society are implicated; they should look to it with a view to correct the evil.

Impotency is another evil produced by onanism, and is sometimes difficult to remove. Dr. Thomas enumerates this as one of the most frequent causes. As there is both general and topical weakness, the indications of cure are, to strengthen the system generally, and the debilitated organs in particular. In order to effect this, the patient must be made to abstain from his solitary practice, unless this is obtained, all remedies are useless. The most useful tonics are the cinchona, or the Sulph. of Quinine, the different preparations of iron, wine, cold bathing, and a generous nutrative diet. Cantharides are undoubtedly the best stimulant in the materia medica for recalling the lost energies of the genital organs. The following remarks of Dr. David Hosack on this disease and the properties of this medicine, are particularly valuable.[45] "Many are the causes which may be assigned for disorders of this nature: the abuse of mercury in the treatment of syphilis and of some other diseases, the unsuccessful management of gonorrhea, the still popular and pernicious practice of using lead injections, neglected gleet, excessive venery, and particularly *onanism*, may be enumerated as the principal. *In this condition of the physical system, the intellectual powers of the patient often largely participate; and few cases, indeed, have stronger claims on the attention of the practitioner than those in which these circumstances, arising from these causes, are united. Too frequently the representations and sufferings of the patient are regarded merely as the phantoms of the mind; and from an indifference both as to the real disease and a want of confidence in the means that may be successfully employed, the most deplorable consequences ensue.*

"'The tincture of lytta,' says Dr. Thomas, 'might likewise be of service if given in small doses.' The truth is, there is not an article of the materia medica used in any individual disease, the value of which ought to be estimated more highly than the lytta, in cases of seminal weakness and impotency when arising from the sources just stated. Though until within a few years its internal administration was pronounced to be almost uniformly productive of dangerous effects, yet it is now fully established, by numerous facts, that the instances in which it disagrees with the constitution are extremely rare, and that when, from unforeseen circumstances or peculiarity of habit, the mischief is produced, it can generally be removed by the readiest and mildest means. Occasionally, indeed, an active antiphlogistic treatment, such as blood-letting, saline cathartics or senna and manna; the free use of diluents, as soda water, barley water, etc. and the warm bath, may be demanded. The claims of camphor in counteracting the action of the lytta do not appear to be clearly established. My own experience does not enable me to recommend it: if camphor relieves the morbid symptoms, so seldom excited by the lytta, it must, I think, do it by its anodyne or sedative properties, and not by any peculiar virtues attributed to it; and, if such be the case, I would much rather depend on the use of opium in small doses.[46] Most generally any uneasy or distressing symptoms from the internal use of the lytta disappear of themselves by ceasing for a while to take the medicine, and that too within twenty-four or thirty-six hours afterwards.

"The lytta is not, as is generally supposed, local in its action, but produces a general excitement; it increases the sanguineous circulation, the flow of urine, and the discharges by perspiration: from its disguised action the whole system becomes invigorated, and this altered state is manifested by an enlivened condition both of the mind and body. The morbid discharge from the urethra becomes altered and assumes a thick and opaque aspect, and ultimately the wonted functions of the body are restored.

"The lytta has been recommended to be given in powder, in the form of pills, and in tincture. The only pharmaceutical preparation which I have employed for internal use, is the last. The tincture seems to be the most agreeable, and, in general, the most manageable form. The extent of the dose depends materially on the peculiarity of the case. Roberton observes, 'it seems an invariable rule that the greater the existing debility either of the general habit or of the generative organs, the greater quantity of the lytta is requisite to effect and keep up the irritation in the urinary passages and in such cases the cure is always more tedious. In those apparently stout, small doses, comparatively speaking, can be taken; while in those whose general health, or whose generative organs only are most morbidly affected, can take the most; and, as they approach to health the doses requisite to keep up the irritation must be diminished, the system and also the generative organs being more susceptible of its action.

"Experience strengthens the preceding remarks of Mr. Roberton, to whom we are so much indebted for his valuable work on the Generative System. The dose of the preparation with which I have generally commenced, is twenty or five and twenty drops three time a day in a little wine, tinctura amara, or water. After the use of the articles a few days, the dose is to be increased to thirty or forty drops, and as often repeated within the twenty four hours. It has happened at times, that on the third or fourth clay, and now and then even earlier, that the patient complains of some little uneasiness in passing water: this, if it does not increase, may be, for a while, disregarded; if the pain becomes severe the remedy must be laid aside until the distress abates, after which it may again be prescribed to the same extent, if not greater, until similar effects are again induced: in this manner the use of the lytta is to be continued. A practical precept must be here enforced, *perseverance* in the *use of the remedy*. The extent to which it may be carried would, unaided by experience, seem incredible. Cures have been affected within a few days; at other times, from peculiarity of condition, as many months or years have been required to accomplish the object in view. But such disconsolate cases as call for this prescription demand all the preserver's skill; yet the great success which has followed this practice justifies the firmest perseverance equally on the part of the physician and patient.

"In a case (a Mr. R———, æt. 27 years,) which came under the care of Dr. Francis and myself, in the month of November, 1816, the lamentable condition to which the sufferer had been previously reduced by the bad management of a neglected syphilis, and afterwards still further by an injudicious use of lead injections of an unwarrantable strength for nearly two years, led him, in a state of extreme mental anguish, to disregard the advice given him, and to seek the termination of his anxiety by self-destruction. With this view, he took nearly six ounces of the tincture of cantharides during the night. Yet no dangerous symptoms occurred: he admitted he felt a degree of warmth throughout his body to which he had been a long time a stranger, and that his mind was less depressed than before the commission of this act of folly. He nevertheless went out as usual the next morning: he after this became persuaded that his situation was not altogether hopeless, and that his constitution, as he said, had still some stamina left to justify hopes of a recovery. He was now induced to take the tincture of lytta in the manner and quantity prescribed: two drachms and a half three times a day united with a dessert spoonful of the tinctura amara; a generous diet was also recommended. Within about three weeks from this period he was renovated, and considered himself an altered man. His virile powers resumed their wonted energy; nor has he in the slightest degree relapsed into his former state of weakness. This is unquestionably a rare instance in which the lytta, rashly taken, and to an inordinate amount, was not followed by any serious injury. It nevertheless proves that the accounts generally given of this article exciting deleterious effects in moderate doses, are not to be received but with the greatest caution. The lytta, like the common spirit of turpentine, the effect of which was once supposed to prove fatal, even in small quantity, experience has now shown, may be taken to an extent our predecessors could not have imagined. In obstinate gleets, after the ordinary vegetable and mineral tonics, the iron and gentian pills, the balsams and terebinthinates have failed, I have also given the tincture of lytta in the proportion of a drachm with a teaspoonful or two of bitters three times a day with permanent, advantage."

"An error of Mr. J. Hunter ought here perhaps to be guarded against. 'I think,' says he, 'I have been able to ascertain the fact that when balsams, turpentine, or cantharides are of service, they are almost immediately so; therefore, if upon trial they are not found to lessen or totally remove the gleet in five or six days, I have never continued them longer."

"The beneficial effects of the use of the cantharides will occasionally speedily follow its administration; but this is an effect which in a majority of cases is the result of a continueance of the remedy for a considerable time."

I shall close this appendix, by adding the remarks of Dr. Rush, which show the importance of a proper regimen, in the cure and prevention of these diseases, and confirms the remarks of Tissot on this point as well as on some others. "This appetite, which was implanted in our natures for the purpose of propagating our species, when excessive, becomes a disease both of the body and mind. When restrained, it produces tremors, a flushing of the face, sighing, nocturnal pollutions, hysteria, hypochondriasis, and in women the furor uterinus. When indulged in an undue or a promiscuous intercourse with the female sex, or in onanism, it produces seminal weakness, impotence, dysury, tabes dorsalis, pulmonary consumption, dyspepsia, dimness of sight, vertigo, epilepsy, hypochondriasis, loss of memory, manalgia, fatuity, and death. From a number of letters addressed to me, for advice, I shall select but three, in which many of those symptoms are mentioned, and deplored in the most pathetic terms. The first is from a physician in Massachusetts, dated September 4th, 1793.

"'The gentleman whose case is now submitted to you is about twenty-five years of age, meagre, gloomy, and restless, has a bad countenance, and a lax state of bowels. He imputes his indisposition to his excessive devotedness to Venus, which he thinks has been induced by a morbid state of his body. He has been married three years, had no connection with the sex before he married, and, although he feels disgusted with his stong venereal propensities, he cannot resist them. I advised him to separate himself from his wife by travelling, which he did, but without, experiencing any relief from his disease. He has earnestly requested me to render him impotent, if I could not give him the command of himself in any other way. I have tried several remedies in his case; nothing has done him any good except the sugar of lead, which I was soon obliged to lay aside, from its producing a severe nervous cholic. Wishing to know whether this disease was not seated in his imagination only, I asked whether the gratification of his appetite was equal to his desires. Dixit, per annos tres, quinque vices se coitum fecisse in horis viginti quatuor, et semper semine ejecto.'"

After giving the two other letters which are already introduced into this treatise he adds.

"But these are not all the melancholy and disgusting effects of excess in the indulgence of the sexual appetite. They sometimes discover themselves in the imagination and senses, in a fondness for obscene conversation and books, and in a wanton dalliance with women, long after the ability to gratify the appetite has perished from disease, or age.

"The remote and exciting causes of this disease in the sexual appetite are,

"1. Excessive eating, more especially of high seasoned animal food. The vices of the cities of the plain were derived in part from their ' fullness of bread;' by which is meant an excess of nourishing aliment.

"2. Intemperance in drinking. Hence the frequent transition from the bottle to the brothel! It is because it is so common and natural, that the former is generally mentioned as an apology for the disease contracted in the latter, by young men, in their applications to physicians for remedies for it. The incestuous gratification of the sexual appetite, which was the first sin that revived in the world after the flood, was the effect we are told of the intemperate use of wine.

"3. Idleness. This was another of the causes mentioned in the Old Testament of the vices of the cities of the plain. It is from the effects of indolence and sedentary habits that the venereal appetite prevails with so much force, and with such odious consequences, within the walls of those seminaries of learning, in which a number of young men are herded together, and lodge in the same rooms, or in the same beds.

"The remedies for this appetite, when inordinate, are natural, physical and mental. They are,

"1 . Matrimony; but where this is not practicable, the society of chaste and modest women. While men live by themselves (says La Bruere), they do not view washerwomen or oyster-wenches as washerwomen or oyster-wenches, but simply as women. But by mixing with the sex, they lose the habit of associating the idea of the sex of the women with a cap or a petticoat. I have known few young men of loose morals, who have attached themselves to the society of the ladies. They not only polish their manners, but purify their imaginations.

"2. A diet, consisting simply of vegetables, and prepared without any of the usual condiments that are taken with them. Dr. Stark found his venereal desires nearly extinguished by living upon bread and water. They revived upon a diet of bread and milk, and became more active by eating six or eight ounces of roasted goose every day, with a proportionable quantity of bread. Persons afflicted with this disease should use but little salt in their aliment. Plutarch tells us, it was avoided by the priests in his day, from its disposing to venery. The birth of Venus from the sea was probably intended to signify the connection between the use of salt and the venereal appetite. In recommending a vegetable diet for the cure of this disease, I would remark, that it is effectual only when it succeeds a full animal diet; for we read not only of individuals, but of whole nations, that live upon vegetables and other simple food, in whom the sexual appetite exists in its usual and natural force. In such persons the appetite should be weakened, by reducing the quantity of their aliment.

"3. Temperance in drinking, or rather the total abstinence from all fermented and distilled liquors.

"4. Constant employment in bodily labor or exercise. They both lessen venereal excitability and promote healthy excitement. Hippocrates tells us the Scythians, who nearly lived upon horseback, were free from venereal desires. Long journeys on horseback should therefore be recommended for the morbid degrees of this appetite. The chase would probably serve the same purpose. The connection between this exercise and chastity is happily illustrated by the poets in the character of Diana, who lived by hunting. The Indians owe the weakness of their venereal desires to this, among other invigorating employments.

"5. The cold bath. There is a debility of body which is connected with venereal excitability, and which the cold bath is calculated to remove. This excitability is most apt to occur during the convalescence, or soon after the recovery from malignant or chronic fevers. Twelve marriages took place of the patients who recovered from the yellow fever at Bush-Hill, in the neighborhood of this city, in the year 1793; and a greater number were detected in a criminal intercouse with each other in the private apartments and tents belonging to the hospital. I have known two instances of young clergymen, who married the women who nursed them in chronic fevers, both of whom were in very humble life. The celebrated Mr. Howard did the same thing. These unequal matches appear to have been the effects of a morbid sexual appetite, that suddenly succeeded their fevers, and which they did not dare to gratify but in a lawful way.

"6. A salivation, by diverting morbid excitability from the genitals to the mouth and throat, would probably be useful in this disease.

"7. Avoiding all dalliance with the female sex. I knew a gentleman in this city, who assured me he had gained a complete victory over his venereal desires by a strict regard to this direction; and I have heard of a clergyman, who overcame this appetite by never looking directly in the face of a woman.

"8. Avoiding the sight of obscene pictures, the reading obscene books, and listening to obscene conversation, all of which administer fuel to the sexual appetite.

"9. Certain tones of music have sometimes suddenly relieved a paroxysm of venereal desires.

"10. Dr. Boerhaave says, a sudden fit of laughter has sometimes had the same effect.

"11. Close application of the mind to business, or study of any kind, more especially to the mathematics. Sir Isaac Newton conquered this appetite by means of the latter study, and the late Dr. Fothergill by constant application to business. Both these great and good men lived and died bachelors, and both declared, upon their death beds, that they had never known, in a single instance, a criminal connection with the female sex.

"12. The influence of an active passion, that shall predominate over the sexual appetite. The love of military glory, so common among the American Indians, by combining with the hardships of a savage life, contributes very much to weaken their venereal desires.

"13. Several medicines have been recommended to subdue the excess of the sexual appetite; among these, the castor oil nut, and camphor, have been most commended. The former acts only by opening the bowels, and thereby taking off the tension of the contiguous genital organs. Any other lenient purge would probably have the same effect. If camphor have any virtues, in this disease, it must be by its stimulating powers removing that nervous debility, upon which venereal excitability depends. Any other stimulating medicine, given in a similar state of the system, would probably have the same, or a greater, effect.

"I have thus mentioned all the remedies for derangement in the passions and sexual appetite. While I admit the necessity of their being aided by religious influence, in order to render them successful, I maintain that religious influence is seldom effectual for that purpose, unless it be combined with those physical remedies. This opinion is amply supported by numerous precepts in the Old and New Testaments, and it is only by inculcating those physical precepts, with such as are of a religious and moral nature, that the latter can produce their full effects upon the body and mind."

NOTES.

1. '*The author of Genesis.*" An epithet for God.

2. '*the crime of Onan.*' In the Book of Genesis, Onan copulated with Tamar and, before he reached the climax, he withdrew. The word 'onanism' has therefore become synonymous with masturbation.

3. '*Galen.*' Galen (129–200) was a prominent Greek physician, surgeon and philosopher in the Roman empire. He is regarded as the most accomplished medical researcher of ancient times and his medicine was generally regarded as true until the time of Paracelsus, Vesalius and other personages.

4. '*Diogenes.*' Diogenes of Sinope (412–323 BC) was a Greek philosopher who founded the Cynic school of philosophy. In his biography of Diogenes of Sinope, Diogenes Laërtius writes that, when Diogenes of Sinope was caught masturbating in public, he replied, "I wish it were as easy to banish hunger by rubbing my belly." Galen did not glean his information from Laërtius, however, since the historian lived in the 3rd century AD.

5. '*Celsus.*' Aulus Cornelius Celsus, after whom Paracelsus named himself. He flourished from 25BC–50AD and is known primarily for his work De Medicina, which is believed to be the only surviving section of a much larger encyclopedia.

6. '*Aretæus.*' Aretæus was one of the msot celebrated of ancient Greek physicians. He practiced during the reign of Emperor Nero. During that time in the Roman empire, Greeks dominated the medical profession, even leading to the Roman poet Juvenal to say some unkind words about the Greeks who lived in Rome and dominated the said practice.

7. '*burgomaster.*' In German, 'burgomeister' literally means the 'master of the borough,' and was an old title for a chief magistrate or chairman of the executive council, usually of a sub-national level of administration such as a city or a similar entity.

8. '*Mémoires des curieux de la nature.*' Memoirs on the curiosities of nature.

9. '*Boerhaave.*' Herman Boerhaave (1668–1738) was a Dutch botanist, Christian humanist and physician of European fame. He is regarded as the founder of clinical teaching and of the modern academic hospital and is sometimes referred to as the 'father of physiology.'

10. '*coccyx.*' The small bone at the end of the spine.

11. '*Onania.*' This is a reference to a 1724 book published in London and entitled, Onania; or, the Heinous Sin of Self-Pollution, and All its Frightful Consquences. It is also a book on masturbation and the manner in which the habit pollutes the mind.

12. '*hypochondriasis.*' Hypochondria.

13. '*dyspnoea.*' Dyspnea. Shortness of breath or breathlessness.

14. '*priapism.*' The potentially painful medical condition in which the erect penis does not return to its flaccid state, despite the absence of both physical and psychological stimulation, within four hours.

15. [This is an original footnote of Tissot.] Rush, in his Medical Inquiries and Observations upon the Diseases of the Mind, page 349, gives the following case, communicated in a letter, by a physician in Virginia. "A. B., aged seventeen, of cold phlegmatic temperament of body, of a sedentary life, and studious habits, in consequence of indulging in the solitary vice of onanism, has lately become very much diseased. His vision is indistinct, and his memory much impaired, and he now labors under much muscular relaxation, prostration of strength, atrophy, and depression of spirits. His system is so very irritable, that the least agitation of mind, or riding on horseback, or gently rubbing his breast, or even combing his hair, produces emissions of semen."

16. '*edematous.*' Relating to edema (or hydropsy), which is an abnormal accumulation of fluid in the interstitium, located beneath the skin and in the cavities of the body.

17. [This is an original footnote of Tissot.] An individual acknowledging the cause to be onanism, writes thus: "I rest badly at nights, and am much troubled with dreams. I have frequent nocturnal erections, accompanied with a sensation of uneasiness, instead of desire or pleasure; and from dreams, frequent emissions take place, which are much more fluid than natural. The external organs of generation have a numb, or dead feeling. The lower part of my back is weak; my eyes are often painful, and my eyelids swelled and red. I have an almost constant cold, and oppression at my stomach. In short, I had rather be laid in the silent tomb, and encounter that dreadful uncertainty hereafter, than remain in my present unhappy and degraded situation." — Rush's Med. Inquir. Trans.

18. '*Rhazes.*' Muhammad ibn Zakariya Razi (845–925) Persian alchemist, physician and chemist and one of the most renowned figures in the history of medicine. He was an early proponent of experimental medicine, the father of pediatrics and a pioneer of ophthalmology.

19. '*syncope.*' Fainting or passing out. A short loss of consciousness and muscle strength, characterized by a fast onset, short duration, and spontaneous recovery. It is due to a decrease in blood flow to the entire brain and from low blood pressure.

20. '*jeu de dames.*' French for the 'game of women.' The phrase means a man attempting to woo women and engage in coition.

21. '*pleuritis.*' Pleurisy. An inflammation of the pleura, the lining surrounding the lungs.

22. '*sacrum.*' A large, triangular bone at the base of the spine and at the upper, back part of the pelvic cavity, where it is inserted like a wedge between the two hip bones.

23. '*fièvre ardente des épuisés.*' This roughly translated into English as the 'strong fever of those who are worn-out.'

24. '*dysuria.*' Painful urination.

25. '*cataplasm.*' Sometimes called a 'poultice.' It is a soft, moist mass, often heated and medicated, that is spread on cloth over the skin to treat an aching, inflamed, or painful part of the body.

26. '*Rachitis.*' Rickets. A defective mineralization of bones before epiphyseal closure in immature mammals due to deficiency or impaired metabolism of vitamin D, phosphorous or calcium, potentially leading to fractures and deformity.

27. '*nervines.*' A plant remedy that is said to effect the nervous system beneficially in some way.

28. '*menses.*' Menstruation.

29. Juvenal, Satires. 6, v. 321.

30. [This is an original footnote of Tissot.] Illas dixit Græcia TRIBADES, Gallis dicunter RIBAUDES: monstrum quotidie nascens et cui eo confidentius sese tradunt puellæ quod abest fœcunditas et ut dixit JUVENALIS: Quod abortivo non est opus.

31. '*Laufella and Medullina.*' Characters in Roman literature. Laufella mimicked a male lover and sought to woo Medullina. It was a lesbian affair and that is Tissot's point in mentioning it.

32. '*huile essentielle.*' In French, this means the 'essential oil.'

33. [This is an original footnote of Tissot.] I adopt here the common opinion that the veins absorb. Admitting Hunter's opinion that absorption occurs only in the lymphatics, the genital parts will according to this theory be adapted to absorption since vessels of this kind are here very numerous.

34. [This is an original footnote of Tissot.] "Dr. Krimer, of Aach, has lately published an interesting paper on this subject. Our own experience has furnished us with several opportunities of seeing cases, of the kind he describes; and as the subject has not hitherto been particularly discussed, we shall give the leading points of his communication. Dr. K. is of opinion, that diseases of the heart, which have increased so much within the last twenty years, do not always depend upon organic alteration, but are very frequently produced by the baneful, and lamentably frequent practice of the vice of onanism. Headaches, great anxiety, palpitations, faintness, an oppression, and unusual sensibility in the epigastric region, are the first symptoms produced. They increase in severity, in proportion, as the subject gives way to the gratification of his unnatural propensity, and quickly diminish, or cease altogether, if he abandons it. To support his opinions, Dr. K. states many cases. He enumerates the following symptoms, as pathognomonic of such affections of the heart; by an attention to which, the practitioner will be enabled to distinguish the train of symptoms from other diseases, which are not unfrequently suspected." (1.) The hair loses its natural brilliancy, is remarkably dry, and frequently splits at the extremities. It falls off easily, and in large quantities, especially from the fore part of the head. In persons affected with consumption, or organic disease of the heart, the hairs appear well nourished, and rarely fall off. (2.) The eyes are dull, downcast, frequently full of tears, and without expression, and deeply sunk in their orbits. The edges of the eyelids are reddish, and surrounded by a bluish tint. In phthisical patients, and those with organic disease of the heart, the eyes are brilliant, and always preserve their natural expression and vivacity. In young females, at the approach of menstruation, a blue circle is commonly observed around the eye, but here also their brilliancy is undiminished. (3.) The patient appears very timid, and unwilling to look other people in the face. (4.) Periodical headache is common, extending from the occiput towards he forehead. (5.) The power of sight is diminished; the appetite is lost; the tongue is usually loaded. A slight cough, short and difficult respiration, are generally present; but still the patient can draw a deep respiration. (6.) Pains in the stomach, with weight and pressure in the epigastric regions. Patients with organic diseases of the heart have occasionally these symptoms; but in such cases, they are not accompanied by those above enumerated. (7.) A general feeling of lassitude, and

feebleness of the limbs, with pains in the lower part of the back. We would add also, that pain and throbbing of the testicles, with uneasy sensations shooting up the spermatic cord, are frequently complained of. (8.) The perspiration has a dull and sweetish odor, similar to at of infants at the breast. (9.) If the vice of onanism be touched upon in conversation, the agitation and embarrasment of the patient invariably betray him. (10.) If the practice be continued, the mind is at length enfeebled, the patient is incapable of mental or bodily exertion, and sinks into a state of somnolency." —Lond. Med. Gaz., Vol. i. No. 19, taken from Hufeland's Journal.

35. '*dyspepsia.*' Indigestion. A condition of impaired digestion.

36. '*marasmus.*' A form of severe malnutrition characterized by energy deficiency. Those with marasmus look emaciated.

37. [This is an original footnote from Tissot.] In tentigine ardentissima juvenum inest quid grati in ore ventriculi, in concubitum si ruant salacissimi, et ultra vires tentant opus, tunc in ore ventriculi manet illud ingratissimum amarumque quod exprimere nequeunt: pœnas et luunt, et pœnitentia dolent: hinc macies, marasmus, etc. G, R, DE PAYVA, de affectu atrabilarjo, rnirachiali, etc, p, 27.

38. The author seems here to allude to the special punishment of Onan. "And the thing which he did displeased the Lord: therefore he slew him also." Genesis 38:10.

39. '*colic.*' A sharp sudden pain in the stomach, or a physical condition in which a baby is very uncomfortable and cries for long periods of time. In this context, Tissot is using the word in the former sense.

40. '*ferinaceous.*' Having a mealy texture or surface. Containing or rich in starch.

41. '*valetudinarian.*' A person who is unduly anxious about their health.

42. 1 Corinthians 6:9.

43. The testicles secrete the semen, and are the most important part of the genital organs, since the action of this fluid on the body of the female can alone cause the formation of a perfect new organism. The component parts of semen in 1000, are, water 900, animal mucilage 60, phosphate of lime 30, soda 10. The testicles also perform an important part in the individual organism; for when they do not exist, or when they have been removed, the body and mind vary more or less from the normal state, the larynx and the voice ate not developed, the beard does not grow; in short, the individual does not acquire the distinctive characters ofnis sex." See the very excellent translation of Meckel's General, Descriptive and Pathological Anatomy, in three volumes, by A. Sidney Doane, M. D. Vol. hi. p. 428, just published. The full and faithful descriptions, the minute details, the systematic arrangement and numerous references which characterize this work, render it one of the most valuable productions on this science in the English language, and ought to be in the possession of every physician.

44. Vol. II. page 155.

45. Appendix to Dr. Thomas' practice. page 1028.

46. See also Orfila on Poisons.

19767596R00113

Made in the USA
Middletown, DE
07 December 2018